You Stuck What in Where?

A Collection of Reader-Submitted Medical Stories

Kerry Hamm

<u>Warning:</u>

This edition features light profanity that may be offensive to some readers. The profanity has been used sparingly and in each instance the usage was included in the submission. I have chosen to leave some of these words in to emphasize portions of the stories.

By now, I am sure you are all too familiar with my *Real Stories from a Small-Town ER* series, which were collections of stories told to you from my time as a registration clerk in Ohio. If you are new here, don't fret! You don't have to worry about a 'certain order' for *any* of my books, including this one!

I have since moved on from the hospital scene, but that hasn't stopped readers from submitting stories of their own experiences from the medical field. Over time, I have received hundreds of stories-some funny, some sad, some downright scary or grotesque-and have worked with my readers to bring these stories to you in a follow up to my last *Real Stories* volume.

If I've learned anything from writing my series and compiling this book, it's that none of us are alone. We're all proof that we've seen some seriously messed up things out there, right? We have seen the good. We've seen the bad. We've seen the downright vile and disgusting. And then, we've seen the humor in these situations and we've been fortunate enough to share them with one another. There is a certain peace in knowing that as no matter how crazy we feel, we have formed solidarity amongst ourselves, knowing that for every bad day you've had, others have had them too. We have worked through the challenges of getting up and facing another drug seeker, another child abuse case, another young death, and another 'how the heck did that even happen?' moment together. You guys are not alone, and this book reaffirms that.

Several of the stories have been edited to bring you clear-cut and clean versions of tales submitted by loyal readers. I have done my very best to edit out hospital and town names, and in some cases my submitters wished to withhold their initials and other details from publication or requested that I edit stories for grammar/spelling. Some stories have been edited for length. I do my very best to preserve a reader's humor and emotions, as well as capture the reader's personality when I edit these submissions.

Though some of the stories in this collection are horrifying, I am glad none of us are alone in what we've witnessed or experienced.

Cheat Sheet

Some readers have been confused about terms used in this series. Here's a quick list to help you out!

LEO: Law Enforcement Officer

ETOH: shorthand for Ethyl Alcohol or Ethanol; commonly used to describe intoxicated individuals

Bus/Rig/Truck: Ambulance

M.D.: Medical Doctor

R.N.: Registered Nurse

MVA: Motor Vehicle Accident

EMS: Emergency Medical Services

EMT: Emergency Medical Technician

PD/FD: Police Department/Fire Department

D.A.: District Attorney

BOLO: Be on (the) Lookout

DCFS/CPS: Department of Children and Family Services/Child Protective Services

SNF: Skilled Nursing Facility. This can be a nursing home or facilities for patients in need of supervised care

AMA: Against Medical Advice

LWBS/LBT: Left Without Being Seen/Left Before Triage

You'll Still Be Here, Right?

It was late in the summer, and I couldn't wait for the season to end. I remember the day clearly, and probably only remember it because I was miserable. Area power grids had become overwhelmed, which knocked out power to about half the city. Of course, my power went out while I was sleeping, so none of my fans or window AC units worked. I took a cold shower, but it was so hot in my apartment that the cold water wasn't much relief. By the time I was ready to leave for work, my scrubs were drenched in sweat, and I hadn't even gone down the nine flights of stairs to get out of the building yet. I grabbed extra scrubs, planning to change at work, where I was scheduled for a 14-hour shift in the ER.

I was about 10 blocks away from my house, when I realized I had forgotten my lunch and my wallet. I figured I could try to bum some cash from my coworkers, just to tide me over on the shift. I remember thinking that I probably wouldn't get much of a chance to eat, anyway, because it was a full moon that night. I've read your stories about full moons in your small town. Honey, come work as a CNA in NYC during a full moon, and you'll see what real chaos is.

Now, you have a feel of how hectic and frustrating my day was going so far. I tried to stay calm, but I always left for work in evening traffic, and I was losing my temper with everyone around me.

Everything happened so quickly.

I remember that I was at a green light and I yelled, "GO!" at the car in front of me. I remember driving forward. I remember being right under the bundle of street signals, and I remember the sounds of horns honking and the smells from street vendor carts. Then, the next thing I knew, I was sandwiched between my seat and the air bag. I couldn't move, except for a light wiggle of the fingers on my right hand. I frantically scanned where my eyes could move; there was blood all over the air bag, and a long strip of metal impaled my left arm. I could see blood running over my skin, but I couldn't feel it. I knew it was bad. I tried to wiggle my toes or lift my legs. I couldn't feel either motion, and I didn't have a way to see if I could do either. At that point, I realized a bad situation escalated to something much worse.

An older woman ran up to my driver's side of my 1994 compact SUV and tried to open the door, but she couldn't. I was in and out of consciousness, but I heard her scream to someone else, "He's a doctor!"

It's so stupid, I know, but I actually remember laughing to myself and thinking, 'I wish,' because I was already panicking about the hospital bills and how I was going to pay them. What if I was paralyzed? How would I pay back my student loans? How would I live? I could barely afford the apartment I had. My car was falling apart, literally—I used duct tape to keep the bumper in place. I couldn't afford to move. I couldn't afford to pay a nurse to help me wipe myself or feed myself or help me with every freedom I took for granted. All those thoughts worsened my situation because my anxiety disorder started up, and suddenly I couldn't breathe.

I guess I passed out, because I woke up in an ambulance, with two medics telling me to stay still. I kept asking if I was going to be able to walk again, and nobody would answer me. My left arm hurt like no other pain I'd ever felt before, but I was *glad* to feel the pain because I knew that was a good sign, even though the metal was still jutting out from both sides of my arm. I felt dizzy, and I passed out again.

When I came to the next time, the first thing I saw was a clock over the room door. It was forty minutes after I should have clocked in for my shift. One of my coworkers came in and started assessing my pain and asking me questions. It was a rushed process and she called out for a doctor three times. The doctor said I sustained damage to my vertebrae, and that I would require surgery. I had limited movement in my legs, and I couldn't feel or move below my knees. I was waiting for a surgeon, but only to remove the metal from my arm. That was determined to have missed major arteries and tendons.

I was informed by an officer that the driver of the bucket truck that had slammed into my car had been hospitalized and would be arrested on DWI charges. Nobody could tell me more because that would violate HIPAA.

As I was awaiting surgery, I asked to use my cell phone to call my mother. I noticed a text message from my boss. Someone had complained that I was late for work, so my supervisor sent me a nasty text message, telling me I was fired and not to bother showing up. Un-freaking-believable. I had never been late for a shift, had never called in sick, and I put up with so much crap around that place. I thought everything would be okay once my boss knew I had been in an accident. I called my mom, and she told me not to worry about anything else, to focus on my own health.

Surgery for my arm went quickly and smoothly, but I looked like the Monster from *Frankenstein*. I was admitted to Intensive Care, and another surgeon was supposed to be on the way, so he could read the scans ordered by the ER doctor. Then, we would discuss surgery. I was pretty loaded from all the pain medication, but I couldn't sleep because I was still panicking about everything. The surgeon came in after a while, and he said I needed to get down to the O.R. ASAP, so the next thing I know, I'm waking up from anesthesia, and my mom is in my room, bawling. I thought that was a bad sign, so I started crying.

Anyway, after two weeks in the hospital, I was discharged and was trying to get my life together. I contacted my boss, since I hadn't heard from her. She said she didn't care why I was late for work, and I had been officially dismissed from my position because I failed to report for my shift, and I did not give 'proper notice' that I would not be available to work. Human Resources backed my supervisor and then told me my hospital insurance wouldn't cover any of my hospitalization because I had been fired prior to being admitted. That sounded pretty illegal to me, but I didn't know for sure, so I kind of just moped around and accepted it because I didn't know any better.

I couldn't believe it. My bills were already piling up. Rent was due, but I couldn't stay at my apartment. I was staying at my mom's house due to mobility reasons. I couldn't return to work because I was ordered to physical therapy and couldn't walk yet. I tried to get a temporary hardship deferment for my student loans, but every person I talked to said my position didn't qualify as a hardship, so I'd have to figure out how to come up with my monthly payment. This had to be some kind of joke.

My mom told me to get a lawyer, so after a few weeks, I called everyone in the phone book. I couldn't afford most of the attorneys I called, and some said they'd work for free upfront, but if I lost my case I'd owe them money, and I could potentially end up owing the hospital money. Ha, *I'd* have to pay *them* for screwing me over? No, thanks. Some of the people I called just sounded sleazy and unprofessional. Finally, though, I found someone to take on my case.

I sued the hospital for wrongful termination and thought I was going to lose because the judge seemed to be on their side. But, in the end, I won. The hospital was ordered to pay me back-pay and a large sum of money as a settlement.

I was in physical therapy for six months before I could walk again, and then I had to use a walker for a few months. I gave up my apartment and lived with my mom for all that time; I don't know what I would have done without her. Now, I can usually walk unassisted, but there are days I have to use a cane. I can't walk for more than a few minutes at a time. Sometimes I have to go to the ER for back pain that the doctors say will never fully go away. I'm in my early-20s.

After my lawsuit, I guess the hospital got hit with a few more—including an investigation of illegal insurance practices. A lot of my coworkers quit. The woman who complained to my boss contacted me and apologized. She said she was having a bad day and didn't realize I had been in an accident. She quit that job, too, and we still talk every now and then.

I don't know what happened to the truck driver. His company's insurance paid for my medical bills and everything. I ended up getting another settlement from that company, just because they were afraid I would take them to court and sue for more. Honestly, I was just glad the company stepped up and was accountable for their employee's actions.

I know it sounds bad, but I'm kind of glad this accident happened. I mean, sure, I'd love to be able to go back to the days when I didn't have scars or mobility issues, back to when I didn't have a handicap placard on my rearview mirror. But, getting in that accident and receiving the settlements helped me financially, and it helped me get a job at a therapy center, helping others recover. I really feel I can help more people this way, because I know what they're feeling, and I know how to encourage them—and they encourage me. I'm much happier in this position than I ever was as an ER CNA.

--J.M.
New York

P.L. from Wisconsin wrote,

"Kerry, my Christmas went well. The cops were called twice, and only four of my family members went to jail. Usually, our family get-togethers are a lot worse."

(I have not received any other messages from this reader, so I'm not sure about the backstory here.)

<u>The Spark</u>

I'm sharing my embarrassing story, so that it will (hopefully) help others make better decisions…or at least be more careful before hitting the send button.

Maybe I should know better, but I like to take racy pictures of myself and send them to my husband via e-mail or text message. I'm not going to lie: in some of my pictures, I'm not dressed, and sometimes I'll get in a sexy position before snapping the picture. I find it really keeps the spark alive in my marriage, and if you've ever been with someone for 19 years, you'll know that you need all the help you can get to keep the excitement from getting squashed by sick kids, unexpected doctor bills, or replacing your son's saxophone because his older brother thought it'd be funny to pour vinegar and baking soda down the horn (I still don't know why he thought it was a good idea, but I do know I had to pay the school for the loaner instrument, and then we had to shell out even more money for a replacement).

My husband's name is John. Well, our house supervisor's name is also John. This super wasn't with the hospital very long at the time, and I had been in a rush when I added his contact information to my phone, so I had two 'Johns' listed in my contact file.

Yes, I'm sure you know what happened.

Well, I didn't know what happened until my husband came home from work. I asked if he liked the multiple pictures of me performing a striptease (which I had captioned with naughty invitations, like, 'I bet you can't wait to be inside me'), to which he replied he hadn't received pictures. He was all hot and heavy, but I was too scared to get in the mood, and as soon as I realized I had texted twelve pictures to the house supervisor, I was so embarrassed and nervous that my stomach became upset and I spent a half hour on the toilet.

As I was suffering from nerve-induced diarrhea, I received a call from my immediate supervisor. She said she needed me to come in an hour before my shift was to start that night. She wouldn't tell me anything else, and she wouldn't listen when I tried to explain the situation.

When I arrived at the hospital, where I work as an RN on the Oncology Hospice floor, I was met by my boss, one of the Human Resources mediators, and two security guards. I vomited in the waste basket, but I still had to attend the meeting.

We walked down to a conference room, and inside the house supervisor was already there, sitting next to another HR mediator and the head of HR, who doesn't *ever* get involved in employee relations unless there's a major code violation or the hospital is being sued for an employee's misconduct. I vomited again and couldn't stop dry heaving, so my boss just told me to bring the waste basket to the table and use it while the HR people talked.

Almost immediately, the HR head said to me that I should know what the meeting was regarding, and he said he was letting me go. He said the house supervisor wanted to file a lawsuit, claiming sexual harassment. The house supervisor said to the mediator that he intended to file the lawsuit, even if I was terminated, and he was going to name me in the suit.

I was sobbing as I explained to the house supervisor that he and my husband shared the same name. I think I vomited three times as I was begging him not to sue me or the hospital. I don't know how many times I apologized, and before I knew it, I was telling the whole room about how my marriage almost fell apart at one point, how long my husband and I were in marriage counseling, and then all about every stressor in our lives. I explained the pictures like I did to you, and I vomited a few more times.

I was sent home and a coworker had already been called to cover my shift. They had told other people that I was fired before they had even called me in. Since everyone knew, they sent texts and Facebook messages all night, trying to find out why I was being let go. I was too embarrassed to reply.

The next day, after a sleepless night and a huge fight with my husband, I received a phone call from my supervisor. She said the house supervisor signed a statement that basically promised he would not sue the hospital for the incident, and that HR would allow me to continue my job, but I would be on a lengthy probation, *after* I fulfilled a one-week unpaid suspension.

I can't tell you how traumatizing this incident was to me, the house supervisor, Human Resources, and my family. My husband and I have agreed to end the racy texts and just surprise each other with lingerie or other things at home. If anyone out there sends stuff like this, make sure you're checking three times before you click that send button! This incident almost ruined my entire life.

--Initials and location withheld at request

<u>Slippery When Wet</u>

Let me tell you about the worse day I've ever had.

During a nasty daytime storm, a tree fell on my house and the roof collapsed. I couldn't use my bathroom or bedroom. I removed what belongings I could, and since I honestly couldn't do more than that, I asked the neighbors to please keep an eye on my house for the night. I'd go to work and have a contractor come out in the morning. I then called work, where I am employed on ICU, and was granted permission to rent a vacant patient room, since my situation perfectly fit our facility's 'disaster policy,' which extended free temporary boarding to employees due to emergencies. I had permission to use the room for five days.

I packed what clothes I could find that weren't wet or damaged from the roof collapse, and I went to work. I took one of the rooms at the end of the hall, which was fitted with a bathroom that was slightly larger than my own bathroom. There was a toilet, a sink, and a walk-in shower.

I hopped in the shower and had just lathered on a heaping handful of shampoo, trying to get the plaster and debris out of my hair, when I had the urge to…well, I had to poop.

Thinking I could 'be really quick' about it, I left the shampoo on my hair, left the water running, and I hurried over to the toilet.

Well, as soon as I sat down, my ass slipped from the toilet seat and I hit the back of my head on the toilet. My tailbone hurt from when I smacked it on the tile floor, and my eyes were burning because the shampoo had run into them.

Two of my coworkers ran in to check on me and I screamed. I realized I had pulled the emergency call chain when I slipped. If you're not familiar with this, it's just a beaded string that hangs from the wall. When pulled, an alarm sounds at the nurses' station. Nurses are required to inspect any emergency alarm as soon as possible.

You'd think that'd be the worst part, right? You'd think that having my female coworkers run in to find me naked, with my penis on show for the world, with shampoo blinding me, with my head bleeding...that's all *pretty bad,* right?

You know what's worse?

Just because I fell off the toilet, doesn't mean I didn't poop. I had explosive diarrhea as I fell, which splattered all over the toilet, floor, and all over my body.

Pretty bad, huh?

That's not even the worst of it.

I tried to stand, but my legs were weak, and I felt extreme pain to my tailbone region. I fell again, and this time landed on my frontal region, so now I was covered in diarrhea, back and front. My coworkers called to the ES and several nurses helped me on a gurney. I sustained a coccyx fracture and was out of work for six weeks.

I sent my coworkers flowers and bought them gift cards to their favorite restaurants. I felt so embarrassed that I didn't know if I could ever show my face at work again.

The good news from all of this, I guess, is that I got my roof fixed. That would have happened, anyway, but I have to find the light in the story somewhere.

--M.O.
Florida

<u>Sweet Dreams</u>

So, yesterday I was diagnosed with a sleeping disorder.

I made an appointment with my hospital's sleep lab, because last week I had an episode where I undressed and walked around naked, while acting out a dream that I was looking for my daughter's lost hamster.

For starters, my daughter doesn't even own a hamster.

Secondly, I was napping in the nurse's lounge when this happened.

One of our doctors found me wandering the halls completely naked. He called for a female nurse to help me get back to the lounge and put my scrubs back on.

That sure made for one hell of the rest of the shift.

--L.K.
Arizona

<u>Priorities</u>

We received a patient with a cardiac history. This gentleman was accompanied to the emergency room by his wife. They were both over the age of 70. Unfortunately, our male patient was experiencing a heart attack and was ordered to be transferred to a hospital an hour away. He would be transferred by helicopter, and he would then undergo an open-heart bypass.

What I found odd about this, is that the patient's wife checked her wristwatch about every ten minutes. As time passed, she seemed antsy. She signed all paperwork, including transfer papers and surgical consent forms.

When the helicopter was about 15 minutes out, I entered the room with several other nurses, and we prepped the patient for transport. We started explaining to the patient's wife how the ride would go, and we explained that she could also travel by motor vehicle, if she felt more comfortable doing so.

This woman acted like I had called her a dirty name or something. She acted offended by all of this and she stated, "I'm not going with him."

"Ma'am," I explained, "your husband is about to undergo a major surgery. You don't want to accompany him?"

The wife then said, "Well, I'd like to, but I already bought a card bundle and reserved a seat at the hall."

I was confused.

"Bingo," the woman snapped at me. "I've already paid for bingo."

The patient did fly out, and no, to my knowledge, the patient's wife did not go with him…because she had a bingo game.

--N.C.
California

Positive Attitude

   Several years ago, a woman was walking her Shih Tzu, 'Annie,' near a Critical Access/Long-Term Care facility in a small town. Coincidentally, this woman had been employed as an RN by the facility for more than half a decade. She even lived only a block away from the facility, which worked for her and the patients to whom she was dedicated. The woman was happy, left with her thoughts about her upcoming wedding, and with spending her time with her precious dog.

   As the RN moved closer, she noticed a large van parked at an odd angle by a wheelchair ramp. When she saw a driver get in the vehicle and start the engine, she believed the driver would back out and leave the parking lot. When the engine revved with a thunderous roar, the RN quickly lifted Annie from the ground and attempted to move up the wheelchair ramp, to allow the driver a clear path to maneuver the van.

In the blink of an eye, the van rolled back and became wedged against the ramp, up to its driver's side door. The RN was knocked down and rolled as the van's bumper made impact, and she frantically called for Annie. As she stood, with Annie's leash still in her hand, she feared her Shih Tzu was trapped under the vehicle.

With her heart racing, the RN rushed to the facility's entrance and pounded on the door. Annie wasn't just a dog, she was family.

Someone opened the facility door and met the RN with a wheelchair.

The driver of the van was unharmed, but the van's passenger sustained a laceration to her head.

On the other hand, the RN sustained bruising to her ribs, several abrasions to her leg and knee area, could not raise her left arm and additionally, it was discovered she had ripped the interosseous membrane between her right tibia and fibula, popping the bones apart.

I know all of this because I am the RN in this story.

As it turned out, Annie walked away largely unscathed by the incident. Two doctors evaluated me in the ER and in the following days, Annie made a fine 'heating pad' for my ribs.

Just about two weeks later, I walked down the aisle—and I did it while wearing an air cast on my right ankle. Thankfully, I could raise my arm by then. I really didn't care what went wrong at the wedding, thanks to the pain pills my doctors prescribed.

I think I may have had a hairline fracture in my tibia, because now I can predict changes in weather—it really gives new meaning to the phrase 'bone chilling cold!'

I've been an RN at the facility for 22 years now.

My heart, Annie, lived for several more years, before succumbing to bone cancer. She was just three months shy of her 16th birthday when she passed in my arms. It did take almost two full years before she could walk by the hospital again, but she spent all her remaining years as her peppy, joyous self and as my best friend.

The best part of the story is that seeing the scars on my leg reminds me of how lucky I am that God spared me, because a few seconds either way could have left me paralyzed or dead. I still get frightened by the sounds of an engine revving up. I cannot wait to see what else God has in store for me!

--S.L.
Kansas

<u>Fate</u>

I was having a scary day. First off, I woke to my three-year-old holding a steak knife about two-inches from my eyeball. He said, "Daddy, hungry," and he dropped the knife. Instinctively, I grabbed it, and I cut my hand.

Downstairs, I was trying to multitask and get breakfast cooked, get the girls' homework checked, sign permission slips for field trips (that were supposed to be brought home two weeks ago, but I'm seeing on the day of the field trip, of course), corral the toddler who acted like he started doing Jager bombs at six in the morning, and get myself ready for work.

I thought, 'Hmmm, I could totally do this. I'll just make fried eggs for everyone, toss in a few frozen sausages, and everyone will be good to go.'

That was, like, two minutes before I left the stove for just a few seconds, and came back to see the pan on fire. As I tried to put it out, I caught my shirt sleeve on fire, and my daughter threw her apple juice on me to put it out. I didn't have time to shower, so I wiped myself off with a wet washcloth, poured the kids cereal, and went upstairs to change. It was a bit disheartening, you know. I'm a doctor. I save lives day in and day out, but I can't seem to manage 'parent life' as well as my wife does (and so simply). My morning was obviously not going well.

In the garage, I tripped over a bike and was almost impaled through the chest by a garden tool. Phew. I started thinking I should call in and hole up with the TV.

Luckily, nothing unusual happened as I was driving the girls to school. Next, I parked across the street from my son's daycare and took him inside. As I was crossing the street to get to my van, a car sped around the corner and almost hit me. The driver hit the brakes, and the car was inches from taking me out.

Okay, this was all a bit much. Someone was sending me a message. I didn't know what the message was, though. Was it a threat? Was it the kind of message to say, 'I can take you out whenever I want,' or was it telling me to be more careful? Whatever the message, I was on edge.

My bad luck continued. I slipped as I was scaling the back stairs to the ER entrance, accidentally slammed my hand in the door, and tripped over a syringe cap that was on the hallway floor.

Okay, someone was trying to kill me. It couldn't have been anything else at this point.

Someone called a code to the third floor, and all available physicians were paged. I thought the third floor was under construction, but I sometimes miss things because I don't pay attention, so I shrugged it off and took off running. The stairs behind the ER can get you anywhere faster than our old elevator can, so I ran full-speed and was out of breath when I pushed open the door to the third floor.

I am not exaggerating about this next part.

As soon as I took about three steps, I fell into a hole in the floor. I don't know how I didn't see it. It was deep enough that I could lie in it, if I curled in a ball. I hit my head on an exposed pipe, and a searing pain shot through my wrist.

All the lights were on. There were no signs taped to the hall door. There were no streamers of tape around the hole in the floor. I mean, once I took a look around, it was clear the unit was still under construction. In the moment, though, I guess I was just focused on the patient than I was at watching where I was going.

I went back to the ER because I was positive my wrist was broken, and an x-ray showed it right there: an intra-articular, nondisplaced distal radius fracture. Someone asked me what happened, and I explained. She replied, "The third floor's been under construction for two months; everyone knows that."

Yeah, well…Turns out the switchboard operator meant to call the code for the *fourth* floor, not the third. But, my bad for not knowing that.

I wish I could say that I went home and enjoyed the rest of my day (at least as well as I could expect), but that's not what happened. As I was leaving the ER, I fell down the same stairs I'd slipped on when I had arrived, and I had to take two staples to the head. I also sprained my right ankle and couldn't drive. My wife couldn't leave work to pick me up, so she called her mother—the same mother who seems to hate me for some reason. For nine years, that nag has been going on and on about how my wife could have married her (mother's) best friend's son and made the two women in-laws, but my wife 'just had to run off and marry the redhead who doesn't eat shrimp—honestly, Jane, who doesn't like shrimp?' (Never mind that I'm highly allergic.)

My mother-in-law refused to stop at the pharmacy for my pain meds (my wife is an attorney and has better insurance than I was offered, so we don't fill our prescriptions at my work), so I had to go home empty-handed and in excruciating pain, especially since most of the meds had worn off since I'd left the ER.

But wait, it doesn't end here!

My mother-in-law 'accidentally' kicked one of my crutches, and I fell as I was hobbling up the walkway. I didn't injure myself again, but it was embarrassing to take a fall in front of the entire neighborhood.

The rest of the afternoon went okay, unless you count the part where my wife brought the kids home and one of my daughters accidentally hit me in the testicles with a ball.

Great day that was…

--P.P., M.D.
Connecticut

I'm Having a Crisis!

If you've ever worked in an ER (or have read any of my books), you know all too well that the department receives more than its fair share of mental health complaints. Here are a few that share a topic that's embarrassing for some people: sex.

I once registered a girl—who'd just turned 18—for suicidal ideations. Her ED nurse said the girl (who still lived with her parents) skipped school and went to an adult bookstore, where she purchased a 'fetish-type' dildo.

As she was paying the clerk, the girl's parents entered the store, saw the dildo, and confronted their daughter about the purchase. The girl tried to lie and say it was a joke, but she also purchased lubricant and some other not-so-kinky toys and accessories. She stated that she and her parents 'got into a screaming match' in the parking lot and the girl drove around for a while, before finally coming to the hospital.

I guess the patient told the nurse that she was too embarrassed to see her parents, and if she had to go home that night, she was going to 'hang [herself] with a belt.'

Since she was 18, she didn't need consent for her visit, and she was admitted as a mental health observation.

--L.W.

Ohio

When I was 15, my mom walked in my room without knocking. I was masturbating and was absolutely mortified to see her standing between my door and my computer desk, where I was seated, jerking off to a DVD I'd stolen from a friend's dad.

At first, I thought the worst part about all of this is that I ejaculated right around the time my mother stepped in.

Well, my mom realized the 'material' playing from the DVD was male-on-male pornography. I didn't get to come out of the closet in my own, unique way or time. I was outed right then, right there.

My mom called the pediatrician and explained 'what had occurred,' by freaking out and saying that I was experiencing a 'crisis.' The receptionist said they couldn't fit me in, and if my mother had concerns regarding my mental health, to take me to the nearest emergency room.

That's exactly what my mom did.

A counselor and doctor sat down with my mom first, and then they took me to a private room and asked me a bunch of questions, like whether or not I felt safe with my mother, if she hit me or abused me in any way, and if I felt my life was in danger before or after the incident. They both said that if I didn't want to go home that night, they could try to get me admitted to a special hospital for pediatric mental health patients.

I told the doctor and the counselor that I just wanted to go home and forget the incident ever happened.

My mom didn't talk to me the whole ride home, and for two weeks she wouldn't make eye contact with me or say much except stuff like, "Your breakfast is on the table," or, "I need you to take out the trash before bed."

I'm in my thirties now, and I have a wonderful relationship with my mom. She's very supportive of my lifestyle, and she adores my boyfriend.

We never really talked about that day, but I think it's safe to say that we both got over it.

--T.V.
Washington

One time, I registered a man who told me he needed to see a doctor because he was having sexual thoughts about his sister. He didn't need to tell me more, but he went on to explain that his fantasies had become more frequent and more erotic, and if he didn't get to talk to a doctor, he was afraid he was going to act on his thoughts and rape his sister.

I've seen a lot of patients, but this one was the worst one ever.

He was admitted, by the way.

--R.D.

New Jersey

My patients were listed on the registration screen as a '2 for 1,' which generally means these patients are family members and are suffering from the same illness, such as a mother and infant. With a '2 for 1,' these patients are placed in the same room and often cared for by one nurse. This cuts down on time and resources.

Some hospitals allow a '2 for 1' for adults, but our hospital does not, so I was curious to know why our veteran registrar signed-in these two patients this way—and for mental health, especially. That's a huge no-no around here.

I walked to the front and was about to confront the registrar, when a woman took a pause from screaming so she could slap a man. Security rushed into the lobby and separated the two.

"Those are your patients," the registrar said to me.

"And what are they here for?"

"Counseling," she said.

"If they're mental health," I asked, "why did you list them as a two-for-one? You know better."

I didn't give the registrar a chance to respond. Instead, I called one of the patients' names. This didn't go over so well, because even though I had called the man's name, the woman who'd slapped him was right at his side, and they immediately started talking over one another to tell me everything about their troubles.

It took 10 minutes in triage before the couple finally said they wanted to see a counselor. Neither was suicidal or felt the need to see a mental health counselor, though.

These people signed into the ER for MARRIAGE counseling, all because the wife commented that the couples' new neighbor was 'yummy,' and to exact revenge, the husband screamed out another woman's name during sex.

Our ER doctor tried to calm the patients, but they argued and argued until they were told the problem did not constitute as an emergency, nor was it a valid reason to meet with a mental health counselor.

--K.R.

New Hampshire

I met with a female patient, regarding a chief complaint of suicidal ideations. The patient, in her late teens, stated she 'needed' to be admitted to the mental health wing, and if she didn't, she 'couldn't go on living.'

At first, the patient refused to explain her mood and/or reasoning behind her threats. It took approximately 30 minutes for the patient to inform me that she had been on top of her boyfriend during sex, when she experienced diarrhea. Realizing what she had done, and being disgusted, the patient then vomited on her boyfriend. He broke up with her and kicked her out of his dorm.

My patient then stated she would kill herself if she had to go back to campus and be faced with the embarrassment.

I allowed the patient to stay on our wing for 24 hours. She checked herself out in the middle of the night.

--S.R.
Florida

One night, at about two in the morning, we received a patient for a suicide attempt. He overdosed on medication.

We learned this patient attempted suicide after he called his new girlfriend the wrong name during sex.

Then, he had to go back and explain who 'Deanna' was.

He was fantasizing about a character from Star Trek.

This guy was so embarrassed that he wanted to kill himself.

It was really sad.

He was admitted.

--M.N.
New Jersey

A single mom brought in her 13-year-old after finding him masturbating in a warm banana peel. She wanted him seen by a counselor because he was 'obviously mentally disturbed' if he was 'having sex with a banana.'

We let the kid sit in the back and watch TV, while one of our male doctors took mom into a different room and told her that the kid was just experimenting with masturbation.

It was crazy there for a while, because she was just hysterical and kept saying stuff like she was afraid her son was going to grow up to be a serial killer because she saw on TV that 'odd sex acts' can be an early sign of 'darkness in your heart.'

Really weird.

--J.T.M.
Maryland

A patient came in one day and spoke broken English. His hand was bleeding profusely and was bleeding through the towel wrapped around it.

"What happened?" I asked, as soon as I saw all the blood.

I could tell he was struggling to find the words. Finally, he blurted out, "Plate take bath!"

We called the translation hotline and learned the man had been doing dishes, when he cut his hand on a knife.

--L.N.
California

<u>Fan Mail</u>

Kerry, I have read every book you've released, and I love them. I am sure this will end up in one of your later books, and I deserve it, because I *just* read about this happening in '*Tis the Season.*

My son thought it would be funny to wrap a heavy gift in 13 layers of saran wrap, so I had to get a knife out to try to cut through all that.

As I made it through the final layer, I kept the knife in my right hand and opened the gift box—it was a large box, so I started thinking my son bought us a new microwave, after hearing that we were having problems with ours.

I opened the box and was met by packing paper—it was the kind that commercial places use, a continuous stream of hard, brown paper all crumpled up on the surface and sides of the box.

I pulled and pulled at this paper with my left hand. It felt like I had yanked 10-miles of the stuff out of the box, and my arm was getting tired. I started using both hands to pull, and I may have gotten a bit excited.

I forgot I had the knife in my hand, until I stabbed myself in the eye.

Our Christmas was interrupted by the need for an ER visit. The knife tip had sliced through my eyelid.

I should have known better. I can't believe that I read about these holiday injuries in your series, and then turned around and stabbed myself.

It wasn't a microwave, by the way. My son taped an envelope under a few weighted bricks. He bought us a cruise.

--K.Y.
Vermont

<u>Dinner Time</u>

I've read all your books and am lucky to say that my hospital doesn't seem to have as many rude patients as you and your other readers have. I also worked as an ER registrar in a small town, and I loved my job. A woman tested me once, though.

This woman, probably in her mid-30s, brought her baby in at 03:30. The baby wasn't fussy, but his mom was.

"How can I help you tonight?"

"*You* can't," the woman snapped. "I need someone who didn't go to college for an arts degree."

(Yes, she really said that. I will never forget those words. I was instantly annoyed at this woman's condescending attitude, but I wasn't offended because I was a second-year nursing student at the time. I was working as a registrar until I could be hired on in the treatment area.)

"Well," I sighed, "you have to register to be seen by a doctor."

"Fine, then do that."

"What seems to be the problem?"

"My baby needs to be seen."

"I can help you with that. What seems to be the problem?"

"Why do I have to talk to you, anyway? Why can't I just see a doctor?"

"Ma'am," I explained, "think of the emergency room as a conveyor belt. We register you here, and your information gets sent to a nurse, who will ask you questions. She'll then give that information to a doctor, and the doctor will diagnose your child."

"Fine, register me."

"Okay, what seems to be the problem?"

"Is this going to take a long time?"

I thought my head was going to explode. I took a quick breath and stated calmly, "As soon as I register you, I'll tell a nurse you're here. But, I need you to please tell me what the problem is."

"You don't have to be so snotty," the woman scolded me.

I apologized for about two minutes straight, still trying to get an answer out of this lady. Finally, she told me her child was refusing food, specifically strained squash.

I thought, 'Are you freaking kidding me? You're going to bring your kid out at three in the morning, just because he doesn't like squash? Seriously?'

I asked the patient to take a seat in the waiting room, and a nurse would be up as soon as one was available. She pitched a fit about that, too.

I wanted to say, "Look, I'm sorry that you just found out that you're not above having to follow the rules like everyone else, but go *sit down* and be mad about it. Don't stand at the desk and stare me down, like I can do anything about it."

I needed the job, though, so I didn't say anything. I pretended to be doing important electronic filing while she stared at me and kept sighing loudly, but really, I was on Facebook, looking at cat memes.

The triage nurse came up front after a few minutes, and he guided the patient's mother to a room just off the side of the registration area. The woman kept staring at me while the nurse asked her questions, and she complained a few times that if I had done my job correctly, she wouldn't have had to repeat her child's problem. I could tell the triage nurse was tired of this woman already.

"So, it says right here," said the nurse, "that your baby is refusing food?"

"Squash, yes."

"How long has he been refusing food?" asked the nurse. I'm not sure that he really thought about the patient's first answer.

"Well, I first tried him on it about three days ago. I've been trying to rotate squash, bananas, and mango as sides. He just won't eat the squash, though. He spits it out."

"Wait," the nurse said. "So, he is eating?"

This question triggered mom.

"If he was eating, I wouldn't bring him in."

"So, he's not eating the bananas and mangos?"

"No, he is."

"So, he is eating?"

"No, I just told you that."

"No," the nurse corrected, "you just said he *is* eating."

"But he won't eat the squash. There's something wrong."

"But…he is eating other food?"

Mom made a growling sound and said loudly, "Is everyone here incompetent? Look, I just told you: he's eating other foods, but he won't eat squash."

"Maybe he doesn't like squash," said the triage nurse. I think he meant to think it , because it sounded more like a stray thought than a statement to the patient's mother.

"That's stupid. There's something wrong. Why am I even talking to you? I want to see a doctor."

"Ma'am," said the nurse, "we're almost done here, and then we can get you to a room. A doctor will see you soon."

"I have insurance. I have real insurance, not welfare. You have to let me skip this crap. I know the law."

"Ma'am," the triage nurse sighed, "everyone must go through the triage process. Well, if you're bleeding to death, we get you straight to a room, but you're not dying, and your son looks like he's doing okay. We're almost done here."

"I'm sorry," the woman shouted, "are you a doctor? Did you go to medical school?"

"I've been a nurse for twenty-three years," triage said dryly.

"But you're not a doctor. You're just a nurse. I want to see a doctor. I want to see someone who's trained to treat my son."

"You know what?" triage asked. "Let's get you to a room. We'll finish these questions later."

Triage got the woman settled in a room, and he back to his office to mutter to himself. I heard him and said, "That one was a peach."

"She said she didn't want to see a doctor who's under the age of thirty, but she also won't be seen by anyone who's older than fifty."

"Seriously?"

"Yeah. She said she wants someone who knows what they're doing, but young enough to understand today's kids."

"What's to understand?" I exclaimed. "That baby's, like, six months old."

"I know. She's crazy. I only took her back because I didn't want to deal with her. I'm marking my questionnaire as an uncooperative guardian."

I think this woman was in back for maybe 10 minutes, before she stormed to the front and approached my work station.

"This hospital is full of frauds," she screamed at me. "Telling me my son doesn't like squash? Won't run any tests because he just ate from green beans just fine? This place is ridiculous."

I started to apologize, but the woman flipped out more.

"I want your name," she shrieked. "I want your name, the guy who made me sit in that room and answer stupid questions and question my parenting, and I want the names of every person just sitting back there, while an incompetent doctor just decided he's going to let my baby die."

I offered to call our house supervisor down, to allow the patient's mother to file a complaint, but she said she wasn't going to waste another second with us because we were all stupid.

The woman called me the next night and every night for a week straight, because her insurance provider denied the claim due to it being deemed 'non-emergent.' She blamed me for this, but that was all on them, because I don't make those decisions.

I'm not angry about her attitude anymore, but I do laugh from time to time, just because she called us stupid and didn't stop to think that *maybe* her kid just didn't find squash palatable.

--G.C.
Georgia

I TRIPLE-DOG Dare You

It was 03:30, and I had just left the 7-11 store, with a hot coffee and a pizza pocket, when I heard screaming and commotion from down the street.

It was colder than a witch's tit outside, but I wasn't exactly on the 'best' side of town, so there were a number of reasons why people could have been out at that time. We receive several domestic violence, assault, property damage, and theft complaints from this area. And well, no matter where I am, if I hear screaming, I'm going to go check it out.

I left my coffee in my cupholder and tried to finish my pizza pocket as I was walking down the block.

As I neared, I witnessed approximately seven males, all of whom appeared to be in their late-teens to early-twenties. They were huddled around a street sign on the corner. I could hear a male was screaming and crying from inside the circle of gentlemen, while the others were in a panicked state. One male stated, "Don't worry, bro. I called 911."

These men were in such a hysteria that they didn't even see me walk up.

"What's going on here?" I asked.

"That was fast," a guy stated. "I just called for help, like, two seconds ago."

I explained that I had heard screaming from down the block.

"It's stuck," a man said hurriedly. "He needs help, dude."

As the crowd moved so I could get closer, I was expecting to see a young man with his tongue stuck to the metal street sign pole.

Not quite.

Did you know, that if you stick the tip of your penis to a metal pole when it's -2 outside, that it will stick?

Because I didn't know that.

Honestly, I never really *thought* about it.

Well, I'm here to tell you that it does stick. Don't rush out to try it. Take my word for it.

Now, I tried to be the voice of reason with these men, but in a rush, two of the stuck-guy's buddies took it upon themselves to 'hurry up and pull' him away from the pole.

Have you ever heard a cat fight? You know that high-pitched yowl that happens, right after a growl?

Imagine a grown man doing that.

As soon as the subject was free from the pole, he passed out.

I ordered the crowd to disperse and radioed dispatch for an ETA on EMS. I expressed urgency due to several factors. It was cold and many of the men had already been complaining about numb extremities. The subject had to be cold, especially with his penis hanging out in the sub-zero temps. His penis was also bleeding from the tip. And, of course, he was unconscious.

EMS transported the man to the nearest ER. I think he was fine, just in shock from the pain. His penis was fine, just some skin missing from the tip.

I never did find out why this guy would whip his penis out in the middle of the night, with everyone around, and stick it to a pole, but I bet that's something he'll never do again.

--I.G.
Michigan

One Last Bit of Excitement

My girlfriend's father died, so I accompanied her to the wake, where her mother was set on playing home videos on a large projector screen to the side of the coffin. I had never been to a wake like that, but it was kind of nice. They had a bunch of video tapes of my girlfriend's father celebrating birthdays, teaching my girlfriend how to roller blade, and those candid family moments, like when you sneak a video of your family member while they're eating or watching TV.

Well, my girlfriend's mom had a breakdown and wanted to watch her wedding video, so I ejected the tape that had my girlfriend's 12th Christmas on it, and I inserted the tape labeled 'WEDDING.'

Some people stood around, watching the video of my mother's girlfriend walking down the aisle, while other people were saying goodbye to my girlfriend's father. All the sudden, I heard a lot of people gasp and exclaim, and I turned around.

My girlfriend's father had taped over his wedding video with him having sex with my girlfriend's mother.

I tried to hurry up and take the tape out of the VCR, but I was freaking out, so I ended up hitting fast forward, then rewind, and then I somehow paused a scene of a blowjob on the screen. I remember screaming, "Who uses tapes anymore? Why wouldn't you put this stuff on DVD?!," and then the VCR wouldn't eject the tape. We had to manually remove the cords that ran from the VCR to the projector.

My girlfriend's mother started sweating, said she felt dizzy, and she sat down on the floor, right there in front of the casket. It took a minute or so to realize she was probably having a heart attack. I was off duty as a tech, so I really couldn't do anything except call 911.

Yes, my girlfriend's mother *did* experience a heart attack. The doctors wanted to admit her, but she signed out AMA because she had to bury her husband.

I feel horrible for laughing, but that was the most screwed up wake I've ever attended. It's sad that my girlfriend's mother had a heart attack, especially at her husband's wake, but the events leading up to that were crazy.

--T.I.
Nebraska

This Old House

My friend introduced me to this hot guy, who suggested we all go 'ghost hunting.' He had a list of 'haunted' houses for us to check out. I think ghost stories are lame, and I don't believe in ghosts, but he was sexy, and I hadn't dated since I found my ex had slept with my sister, so I was eager to impress this new guy.

Well, we found this house way out in the country, and it looked like it could fall to the ground at any moment. It didn't seem like a smart idea to go poking around. Like I said, though, I thought the guy was amazing, and I would have probably chopped off my finger if he asked me to (okay, maybe not that far).

My friend and her boyfriend went investigating in the basement, while the cute guy and I went to the second floor. I was so scared as I climbed the stairs. Everything in the house was covered in dust. There were rats and bugs scurrying all over. Some furniture had been left behind, and it looked old, like maybe from the early-1900s. I'm no furniture expert, though, so I'm not sure how old the stuff was.

Anyway, the cute guy said we should investigate and then call for each other if we found something, so he went down the hall and was talking to the 'spirits,' saying stuff like, "If you're here, give us a sign."

I thought he was a total dork at that point, but oh well. We all have our flaws.

The Big Gulp I had earlier hit me right in that moment, and I couldn't hold it anymore. I found a nasty bathroom and figured it was still better than trying to pee in the bushes out back, so I hovered over this disgusting old toilet and peed. I got a Charlie horse in my thigh and had to sit down for a minute, so I cringed and sat—it was just going to be long enough for the cramp to go away, and then I was going to pull up my panties and jeans.

I can't even lie about this. I have the worst damn luck ever.

When I sat down on the toilet, I heard a loud crack, and the toilet fell through the floor. It crashed in the kitchen and busted into a thousand pieces. Of course, I screamed, because I had been on the toilet.

My crush came running to the bathroom and yelled "Oh my God, did you see an apparition?", only to find me stuck between the first and second floors. My jeans and panties were around my knees, and my shirt had gotten caught on a pipe and was pulled up over my nose, exposing my ratty old t-shirt bra.

And then I fell and felt my ankle snap. I was in so much pain from that, that I didn't realize I couldn't feel my hand. I also broke my wrist. We were all cited for trespassing, so I had to pay a $213 ticket, on top of the medical bills that totaled more than I make in a year. (Thankfully, the hospital worked out a payment plan, so I only owe half of the original total. But, I'm poor, so I'll probably be paying on those bills for the rest of my freaking life.)

The cute guy came to visit me in the hospital and I confessed that I only went to that house because he wanted to, and I wanted to impress him. I asked if he wanted to get together after I healed. I blurted out that we could have sex.

And then he told me he's gay.

--S.M.
Idaho

Au Natural

I am an Emergency Services physician, contracted by a network of facilities in three states. I travel constantly and live out of hotels in areas where I do not have a rental home. I rarely have time to myself, because most of my visits are for only a few days at a time. For example, I was once in Biloxi for 36 hours, with eight-hours to sleep over that time. Then, I traveled to Atlanta, where I was contracted to an ES department for 24 hours.

I was needed for two weeks at one location, and it was like a vacation for me because I had every other day off, and I only worked four-hour shifts on my days on, unless I was paged.

I decided to go to the mall, just for some downtime. Maybe I could go catch a movie afterward. I had all the time in the world.

Every mall I visit, I see these women in a center kiosk performing makeovers. I usually don't have time for makeup, but I wanted to see what these ladies could do for my plain-Jane appearance, so I stepped up and asked for a makeover.

That day, I learned that these ladies typically only do half of your face. That's the catch. You can either wipe off the makeup they put on, or you can walk through the mall looking like that Two-Face guy from *Batman*. My face was a little itchy, but I looked good. There was no way I only wanted to look that good on one side of my face.

I was going to have the ladies finish the other side of my face, but I was paged with not one, but **nine** 911 traumas. A bus and semi had crashed, and there had been fatalities. All physicians, surgeons, life support specialists, and emergency personnel were needed. I had to go.

You could probably imagine the looks I got as I was literally sprinting through the full mall on a weekend, with only half of my face made up. Teenagers were laughing and recording me. Adults were dodging me, surely thinking I was insane and on a rampage.

I jumped in my rental car and sped away.

About two minutes after driving away, I started feeling…different. My face felt numb, and my chest felt tight. Within seconds, I lost control of my vehicle, right as I realized I was in anaphylactic shock.

Another motorist stopped and checked on me. He called 911, but he was told an ambulance would get to us 'as soon as they could find an available unit.' I can only assume a higher power was looking out for me, because the motorist had a peanut allergy and carried an Epi-Pen. He offered to drive me to the hospital.

I had to wait an hour before I could assist with patients. Unfortunately, by that time, three of our traumas had expired. I don't know if my participation would have made a difference. I wonder daily.

It turned out that I was allergic to the 'natural' key ingredient in the makeup the ladies used. I shudder to think what would have happened if they had finished my whole face.

--M.W., M.D.
Traveling Physician

<u>Eek!</u>

Our hospital has a strict no-resting policy, except for our contracted physicians, who also get paid beaucoup bucks to basically sit back and let us (RNs and non-contracted physicians) do all the work. Our administrators are jerks, too, because they think it's perfectly okay to schedule us up to 28-hours for shifts, with no breaks. They get around this by saying we're not in the medical transport field. Lawsuits have been filed. People have quit. It's a mess.

Anyway, most of us in the ED support each other. If we reach that point where we *must* lie down, we hand off our patients and find a place to nap.

I was up with my kids during my time off work, and then I was scheduled for a 19-hour shift. In 15-hours, I'd only eaten a granola bar, drank half a Coke that I found in my working area, and I was dying for a nap. I told my coworkers, and someone said the hospital had closed off the rehab/PT wing for updates, so everyone had been going down there to nap. That sounded like a great idea, and it seemed to be as soon as I stepped in and saw the plush blue mats and actual pillows—sterilized and wrapped in plastic—ready to be used.

I don't know how long I was asleep, but it was a deep sleep. I needed it, I really did.

I must have been really out of it, because I felt my dog licking my face, and when I reached up, I rubbed her head.

It was at that moment that I started to come out of sleep, because I noticed my dog's head was awfully small.

I opened my eyes to see two rats…not mice, RATS, on my chest. One was sniffing and licking my cheek and licking around my lips.

Boy, oh boy. I jumped right up and forgot that I was on a platform physical therapy table. I thought I was just putting my feet over the side of a bed and on the floor, but I fell about two feet, and when I landed, my ankle gave out and I fell to the floor. I hit my head on a 10-pound weight disc.

The rats didn't seem to care at all. One followed me and bit my hand so hard that I was bleeding. I tried to run out of there, but my ankle hurt so bad, so I was hobbling and screaming bloody murder. I didn't even realize I had busted my head open on the weight, until someone peeked down the hall and shouted to someone else that I had been 'beat up by someone.'

You know what? The rat that bit me was STILL chasing me down the hall! I didn't even know rats were that aggressive until that night.

I was almost fired for sneaking into the wing to nap. My coworker lied for me and said I accidentally drank her tea, which contained medicine that made me drowsy. That's the only reason I didn't get fired. I was written up. My supervisor was pissed because I filed workman's comp. The hospital said they weren't going to pay, so I had to get my Union involved, and they threatened to sue the hospital.

We later found out the wing wasn't closed for 'updates.' It was closed because the wing had a rat infestation.

Good to know, way after the fact.

I didn't break my ankle, just a nasty sprain that I made worse by trying to run on it. I closed the gash on my head with glue from a cart. I've had nightmares about rats since this happened.

--L.N.

Location withheld at request

The weirdest foreign body I have extracted from a vagina was a marshmallow. To be clear, I actually removed 27 full-size marshmallows. I won't even describe to you what they looked (or smelled) like, after they were in my patient's vagina for four hours on a summer afternoon.

I didn't ask why she would do something like that. I was too grossed out.

--C.S.
Georgia

Thanks, Pop

I'm going to be honest with you in this submission. I'm not proud of myself, but what's done is done.

My job laid off about 60% of its workforce and moved headquarters overseas, so I've been temporarily living with my parents until I can find another job that paid as much.

My girlfriend and I have had a tumultuous relationship since I lost my job and couldn't afford my apartment. We'd had a bad fight the week before, so I was surprised when she asked to come over to 'make up.'

I met her at the door and walked her upstairs, to my room.

Just as we were going in my room, my dad walked out of the bathroom (shirtless and with a beer in his hand) and said to my girlfriend, "Oh, hey. I'm sorry I walked in on you guys yesterday. I'm so embarrassed."

A demon rose from hell and took over my girlfriend's body at that exact moment.

My dad was already halfway down the stairs, when my girlfriend stared at me and angrily said, "I haven't seen you in a week."

"I know," I answered.

"So," she demanded, "who'd he walk in on?"

I told my girlfriend the truth. Since we'd been fighting, I kind of started looking elsewhere. It was unintentional at first, but I kind of hit it off with a girl I met when I went to turn in a job application. We went out for coffee, and then everything kind of snowballed. I brought her home (when I thought my parents were at work), and we had sex. I didn't know my dad had called off work that day.

I'll tell you something, in case you're ever in this situation.

If your girlfriend finds out you're cheating on her, try to keep her away from your pocketknife collection, okay?

My girlfriend snatched a knife (that my grandfather had given me before he died) from my dresser, and she stabbed me in the arm and thigh, like three times each. I was bleeding all over the place. My dad is hearing impaired, so he couldn't hear me as I was calling for help.

I think my girlfriend would have stabbed me a couple more times, but she got real weird in the middle of her freak-out. She threw the knife on my bed, straightened up, and said calmly, "You know what? I can do better than you."

And then she left. No, "Oh, sorry I stabbed you," or, "Holy shit, I'll call you an ambulance," or, "Please don't call the police." She literally calmly walked away and never said anything else.

I had to call 911 because there was so much blood that I thought she'd hit an artery or something, but the hospital said I got 'lucky.'

My nurse said she was required to contact law enforcement, but when officers showed up, I lied and said I stabbed myself. The cops knew I was lying, but I figured I was the asshole who cheated, and even though she shouldn't have stabbed me, I caused her to fly off the handle like that.

I had to get a total of 32 stitches, but I still had insurance from my old job, so I really didn't have to pay much (money, anyway) for the incident.

My girlfriend—ex, I should say—left me a voicemail saying that she was sorry for 'hurting me,' but she hoped I'd learn from the incident. I haven't heard from her since then.

--Initials and location withheld at request

I checked in a woman who was between 15 and 25-weeks pregnant. She said she was tired of watching all her friends party when she 'wasn't supposed to' drink, so she was going to get drunk. She said she'd read on an alcohol label that drinking alcohol while pregnant could result in stillbirth, birth defects, or miscarriage.

She registered in the ES because she wanted to know if that meant she would be the one who'd be affected, or if the baby would be affected.

--C.C.
Illinois

<u>Drunken Regrets</u>

In the late-1990s, when I was in college, I went to a baseball game with my friends. It was just a minor-league team at a crappy stadium, with maybe one guy selling stale popcorn and probably about 250 people there. The one good thing is that they were selling beer—cheap beer. My friends and I were plastered by the end of the first inning.

I had to take a piss, so I went on an adventure to the bathroom, which was basically a cement room filled with three toilets (with no doors on the stalls) and two urinals on the other wall.

I can barely stand up straight, but let's take a piss at the urinal, right?

I unzipped my pants and (again, I was really drunk) let them drop to my ankles. I moved closer to the urinal.

And there was a rattlesnake, curled in the urinal's basin.

It already wasn't a happy rattlesnake (are there happy rattlesnakes?), but it *really* became upset when I thought pissing on it would be *hilarious.*

The thing bit me. It lunged and sank its fangs in my upper inner thigh. I remember a guy came in right as I was falling back. I also remember that I was so freaking stupid that I was laughing.

Thankfully, the guy who walked in took off his shirt and threw it over the snake before running to the payphone outside and calling 911. I think the snake got away, but the guy who called the ambulance saw it and identified it.

By the time I was admitted to the ER, my thigh was black, I was bleeding and swollen, and I kept passing out. I really don't remember much of the ER admission.

They had to give me 32 vials of antivenom, I was up on an intensive care room for six days, and I had so many nurses and doctors inspecting my package that you'd think my penis was a tourist attraction. I was told I was lucky that I didn't have to have my leg or penis amputated, since the bite was so close to my groin.

My parents were loaded, so thankfully the bill was paid off after a few years, but it came to about $90,000. My mom acted like it was a 'sign from God' and got real clingy. My dad seriously punched me in the mouth the first day I was home from the hospital, and he told me I was stupid. He didn't talk to me for two months, and at one point, he was so mad that he removed me from his will.

Health-wise, my leg has never looked the same. I started suffering from penile dysfunction right after the bite, both when urinating and operating sexually. That's a little embarrassing.

Now that I'm 'grown up,' I can recognize the severity of what happened. I've seen some stories online, where people have posted their hospital bills, and other people have been quick to call the bills fake. I can tell you that getting bitten by a rattlesnake really is something that can bankrupt you, so as if nature hasn't done enough to warn you to stay away, listen to me and stay as far away from these snakes as you possibly can. I'm thankful that the universe didn't kill me off for being a smart-mouthed, stupid, drunk-off-my-rocker college twit.

--Anonymous at request
Arizona

<u>Wipes</u>

A developmentally-disabled mother brought in her newborn baby. The baby, only a few days old, appeared to have chemical burns on most of its body. As expected under these conditions, the baby was screaming constantly, which was the mother's chief complaint. She said that nothing she did made a difference, that the baby would not stop crying. She was also in tears and said her boyfriend told her to make the baby stop crying, or he would kill the child. The mother's arms were covered in bruises and burn marks. She stated her boyfriend and his mother put out cigarettes on her skin and hit her multiple times per day. This woman stated she didn't want to go home because she didn't want her boyfriend to hurt the baby, and that she thought the baby was sick because it was crying.

Before we even realized what was happening, we called Family Services, the police department, and a charity organization that specializes in domestic abuse cases.

We asked mom if she could tell us what laundry detergent she used, asked if she'd bathed the child, asked if she'd used ointment…Mom reached in her diaper bag and pulled out a container of bleach wipes, the kind of disinfectant wipes I use to clean my kitchen counters. She had been using the wipes to bathe the child, wipe formula from the child's face, and as wipes during diaper changes.

This woman had no idea that something she had done had caused harm to her child, and when we explained, she first seemed confused. She said, "But my book said I needed wipes."

When we explained that there are wipes made especially for infants, and that the wipes she was using caused the chemical burns, the mother had an emotional breakdown and started hitting herself in the face.

Family Services took custody of the baby and placed the child with a foster family until a hearing. The domestic violence organization helped the woman relocate to a shelter, but she could not find work due to her disability, so she had a long road ahead of her.

The last I knew, the woman was living in low income apartments and had gotten a job retrieving carts at a grocery store. I don't think she was able to regain custody of her child. I won't judge her because I think she honestly thought she was properly caring for her child, and that's more than I can say for a lot of kids/parents we see in our department.

--O.S.
Illinois

<u>You Never Know</u>

Way back when, we responded to a 911 call reporting an assault and rape. The victim could not speak; a passerby found the victim in an empty parking lot, and the victim gave written testimony. She stated her assailant choked her from behind and pulled her jeans down as she was leaving her salesclerk job for the night.

The victim struggled. She was no match for the assailant physically. Her attacker forced her to the ground and penetrated her. The victim stated her attacker seemed to take pleasure in slamming her head against the parking lot as he raped her.

Luckily, the patient was able to reach the new pepper spray she carried. She stated that when the attacker realized she was holding this, he punched her repeatedly (resulting in a broken jaw). The victim sprayed the assailant across the eyes with the mace, and only then did he finally move off her. Unfortunately, he did not seem to react to the spray. This is not all that uncommon. Some people seem 'immune' to pepper sprays or stun guns.

The victim stated her assailant 'poured globs of sanitizer on his hands' before attempting to insert the sanitizer into her vagina. She kicked him in the leg, and when the assailant saw lights from a nearby vehicle, he ran.

This case hit me hard. My wife experienced something similar when we were dating (about 20 years before this story took place). She was embarrassed that she was raped, and she abruptly ended our relationship and started drinking at home. She never left her house. Her parents and friends were worried. She felt that what happened was her fault, that no man would ever be able to love her or find her attractive, and she was so scared that it would happen again that she dropped out of college because she couldn't continue her education at home. It took a great deal of counseling and constant reassurance to convince my girlfriend to be my wife.

The victim in this case reminded me so much of my wife. I was worried she would react in the same manner.

A few hours later, my shift was ending. I was stressed out, to say the least. All the night shift guys were coming in, and I didn't say more than two words to most of them.

One guy, the troublemaker who'd been on with us for about a year, approached my desk and started thumbing through my reports.

I snapped on him because he wasn't a good officer. He wasn't even a good person. One time, he stopped a pedestrian and arrested the man for public intoxication. That man had been two houses away from his own, after walking two blocks from the pub. He didn't want to drive drunk. The officer in question didn't care. There had been numerous civilian complaints against the officer, and it was clear he enjoyed abusing power. He didn't have many friends in the department, and we had been bugging the department to dismiss him. We were short on officers as it was, though.

"I'm just looking at these gadgets," he said innocently, trying to turn it around on me and make me the one in the wrong for him fidgeting with my case files and items.

He lifted a UV light and asked, "What's this, a light saber?"

I glanced up. He was holding a UV wand that we used to scan scenes for bodily fluids. They were new to our department, and we'd never used them before that night. That should give you an idea of how long ago this case took place.

I explained this to the officer, and he started waving the wand around like he was sword fighting.

"Just put it down," I ordered.

He was quoting Star Wars, when he accidentally pressed the power button. UV light shined over his face.

It was right then that I told the officer that I wanted to question him regarding a case I'd handled that night.

See, the pepper spray the rape victim used was new to the market and was recommended by law enforcement for one simple reason: its residue was visible under UV light.

After a good while, the officer slipped up and we were able to determine he was our assailant, both by his verbal slips, spray residue, and a bruise on his leg—right where the victim stated she kicked her attacker. The officer lawyered up immediately.

This man was sentenced to a maximum-security corrections facility. I don't know what happened to him over the years, and I don't typically interact with victims (especially victims of sexual crimes—that would be inappropriate, in my book), so I don't know what happened to the victim.

This just goes to show that you don't always know who you're working with, but if you have a gut feeling about someone, you should really give it some consideration.

--Initials and location withheld at request

<u>Reaction</u>

I was terminated from my job as an ED scribe because I vomited.

Well, that's not the full story.

The doctor asked me to stand by his side as he examined the patient. He wanted me to take my typical notes (patient's appearance, skin tone, etc.).

When he lifted a roll on the 600-lbs. patient, the sight and smell of the mold growing in the patient's fat folds made me feel ill. I tried to leave the room, but I vomited on the floor.

The doctor said I reacted unprofessionally and that I had no business in 'his' ED. He filed a complaint against me with my supervisor and HR. I'd been there a year, but I'd never seen anything so disgusting.

--A.P.
Iowa

Port-a-Potty

If you're in EMS, you know you and your partner(s) become so close that you may as well be family—except you like each other more than you like your real family. Seriously, though, we're with our partners for some 40-70 hours each week. We have to trust each other with not only our patients' lives, but also our own. You get to really know a person after you've both been awake for 37 hours.

Well, sometimes your shifts aren't so great, say, if your regular partner is placed on a different bus, and you're stuck with the new guy who kind of smells like cheese and wants to have a Barbara Streisand album marathon while you're staging.

After a three-hour staging and listening to *'Papa, Can You Hear Me?'* seven times in a row, we were called across town to an office building fire with injuries and smoke inhalation.

When we got there, all our patients refused ER transport, so that was awesome. The scene wasn't as bad as initially thought, so most of us were sent back to staging or typical runs.

My stomach began hurting as we were leaving, and I hoped I hadn't come down with the bug that was going around the station. I hardly ever get sick, so I'm a huge baby if I ever do get sick. The last thing I wanted to do with my upcoming weekend off was be sitting in front of the toilet, puking and crying.

Traffic was horrendous, and I mean it was the kind of traffic where you want to scream and cuss, then you have one minute where you hope nobody's hurt ahead of you, but then you go right back to being angry because you've been waiting in this huge three-lane bumper-to-bumper mess, just to move half an inch in that time. To make it worse, we were stuck in a tunnel that ran under the bay. I couldn't even use my cell phone to distract myself from my partner's annoying rant about Barbara Streisand vs. Bette Midler.

My stomach hurt even more, and I knew what was coming.

I had to poop.

There I was, this bored girl stuck in a tunnel, no toilet in sight, and I knew what was about to come out of me wasn't going to be good.

There was no light at the end of the tunnel, literally. We were so far from the exit that we couldn't see how much distance we had to get out. The cab was dimly illuminated by these pale-yellow lights in the tunnel.

"I'm going to get sick," I blurted out.

My new partner got mad because I interrupted him. He just shrugged and said, "Just open the door and puke."

"Not that kind of sick," I said.

He laughed and said, "Well, you have to hold it."

"I can't," I said.

I could feel the sick inside me about to come rushing out.

I didn't know what to do. I'd never been in this situation before.

In a moment of panic, I started unbuckling my belt and moved to the back of the bus.

"What are you doing?" my partner screamed.

"I'm going to be sick!" I yelled back.

I didn't know what else to do, so I opened the small red biohazard bin where we put bloody rags and stuff, and I sat on it like a toilet.

The whole time, diarrhea was shooting out of me, the guy up front was singing along with Barbara Streisand at the top of his lungs. I tried to tell him to shut up, but as I opened my mouth to scream, I vomited on the floor…as I was still pooping.

My new partner was super grossed out, and I don't blame him because I was, too. The worst part was I had to use the bin two more times before we got out of the tunnel, and we didn't have enough stuff on us (because apparently my partner neglected to do the supplies check that he was supposed to do) to clean up the puke, so I had to sit in back with vomit rolling back and forth as we drove.

The new guy told my boss all about what happened and said he never wanted to work with me again. My years-long partner was at the station when we made it back, and he took pity on me and cleaned everything up. I spent the whole weekend dying at home.

--K.M.
Virginia

My girlfriend is a nurse, so when I woke up and noticed a rash on my penis, I took a picture and texted it to her, with the caption, 'What does this look like?'

My girlfriend's mother, who I quickly realized I sent the picture to, responded, 'It's not big enough to tell.'

It ended up being an allergic reaction to the lubricant my girlfriend and I had used the night before.

So embarrassing.

--T.Z.
Indiana

I filed a formal complaint against our new ES physician tonight. He accidentally sewed the webbing of a patient's toes together because he was too busy checking out his reflection in the mirror. He blamed me for not telling him that he was making a mistake.

My bad, I didn't know, "Doctor X. Doctor X. DOCTOR X!" wasn't 'trying to tell him.'

--Initials and location withheld at request

Family Turmoil

We received a patient between the ages of 7-9. He was out with friends, when he was hit by a motorist. The child's friends left the scene, and the motorist called 911.

This patient wasn't in critical condition, but he was pretty banged up. He had two broken legs, a broken arm, a concussion, and he had broken two fingers. As a child, he handled the situation better than most adults. Still, however, he was alone and afraid.

The child fell asleep before we could ask more questions, so we went through his cell phone to find his parents' phone numbers. We called his mother first.

I called his mother, and the phone rang 12 times, before it picked up and hung up. I figured this was because I was calling from the hospital, not the child's phone (it was in horrible condition, so much that we were lucky to get the numbers from it). I made another call, and it rang and rang.

Finally, a male picked up.

"What do you want?" he demanded.

I identified myself as a nurse and explained I found the number in the patient's phone. I asked if the child's mother was home, and I stressed that it was an urgent situation.

He set the phone down, and I could hear talking in the background.

"Hey," he said. "Some bitch is on the phone. She said she's from the hospital."

"So?"

"She said she got the number off John's phone."

"So?"

"So, she said she wants to talk to you."

"Well, I don't want to talk to anyone. Take a message."

"I don't want to talk to her again. She sounds like an ogre."

(I lived in the Scots region until I was 23, and I have the accent.)

There was a bunch of cussing and some screaming, before a woman got on the phone and asked with an irritated huff, "Hello?"

"Ma'am," I explained, after verifying she was the child's mother and then introducing myself, "your son was in an accident."

"And what do you want me to do about it?"

"Uh, excuse me?" I asked.

"What do you want me to do about it? I don't have money. Call his dad."

"Uh…"

"It's not that hard to understand, or can't you get that through your head? Call—his—dad."

I read back the number I had for the child's father, to which the woman on the line scoffed, laughed, and said, "I don't know why that number would be in the phone. Johnny Sr. just got a new phone number this morning. Oh, he probably didn't give the number to John. Why would he? He never gave a damn about anything else. Everything's always my responsibility, always my fault. Even tried to tell me it was my fault that he lost his job.

Said I came in there screaming too much and they fired him. Uh, it was a bank. Nobody gives a [eff] if you go in there to talk with someone. And you know what? Who cares if they did care? I'll do whatever the hell I want. Screw them."

"Ma'am," I said cautiously, "do you have another phone number I can try?"

"Baby," I heard the first man say in the background, "want a bump of this? Oh man, this is some good shit."

I am not even kidding. The woman put the phone down, and I could hear someone snorting in the background. I think they were doing lines of cocaine.

"Hello?" I asked loudly. "HELLO?"

I was talking so loudly that my coworkers and other patients were staring.

The woman finally came back to the phone, after about five minutes. She was laughing and seemed…distant.

"Uh, hello?" she asked. It was like she was talking to herself. "Like, holy shit, did I just leave the phone on? Was I going to call someone?"

"Ma'am," I said firmly. "You're still on the line with your son's nurse. Can you give me his dad's phone number or not?"

"You don't have to be such a cunt," she screamed hysterically. "I'll give you the [effing] phone number!"

Uh…

The woman transferred the phone to her male friend, and I could hear her crying and saying, "Just tell her the number. I don't want to talk to her; she's mean. No, just give her the number. I don't know, I thought I wrote it down somewhere. Check the hamper. Sometimes I put paper in the hamper."

I was really hoping the child was never present for those conditions.

It took about 25 minutes on that call, but I finally got another phone number, and I placed that call.

It rang and went to a voicemail (that wasn't set up) three times, before a male answered snippily, "Hello?"

"Sir, is this Johnny Sr.?"

"Look, whatever I owe, I'll pay when I can."

"Sir."

"I don't know what you guys want from me. I'm still paying a divorce lawyer, that bitch gets most of my paycheck in child support, and then I still have to turn around and buy the damn kid everything. You'll get your money when you get it. Leave me alone."

I called two more times before the man answered again.

"I'm going to report you for harassment," he warned.

"I'm from the hospital," I said in a rush. "And I have your son here."

"It's not my week with him. I'm not dealing with this shit."

"Huh?"

"Call his mom."

"But—."

"Call his [effing] mom," the man screamed.

He then hung up on me.

Instead of calling the child's mother, I called DCFS. A caseworker came to the hospital and started a report. She asked the patient some questions and tried to call both parents—with the same results I had.

She then requested the police department send officers to request the parents come to the hospital, hoping this action would prove the severity of the situation. The patient's mother and her boyfriend were arrested because they had drugs in plain sight when they answered the door, and the son's father wasn't home. An officer stayed at the father's residence for three hours, but the man never came home. He was thought to be at the library, where his ex-wife said he worked as a custodian. He wasn't there either. (We later learned he was purposely avoiding being at work or home; he didn't want to be bothered on his 'week off' from his kid.)

DCFS noted the child had been subject of investigation several years earlier, so they tried calling the last guardian he was placed with: his grandmother. Luckily, that phone number was still active, and she stated she would be flying out as soon as she could reserve a seat. She requested that we not return the child to either parent and said she'd been contacting DCFS for more than six months, trying to convince the agency that both parents were guilty of drug abuse and neglect, but the caseworkers she'd spoken with had told her there was no evidence and therefore, they couldn't conduct an investigation.

The boy was transferred to Peds, and I stayed the night. I slept in a chair in his room, just in case he woke up and was scared. I can't have children of my own, so I'll admit I do get a bit too attached to my pediatric patients. I've actually put in a transfer to the floor, but they never have any openings.

DCFS and the child's grandmother went to an emergency hearing soon after, and the grandmother was given temporary full custody of the boy.

You know what?

His parents didn't show up to that hearing, either.

--O.P.

Location withheld at request

I needed my wife to help me with remodeling the garage, so I held plywood to a frame, and she was in charge of using the nail gun, just until the plywood was secure enough not to fall. My wife got too close to my hand and almost put a nail through it.

I jumped back and was cussing so much that I tripped over my toolbox and landed on a board…and impaled my hand on the nail running through the board.

Very expensive four-hour trip to the ER.

--W.U.
Wyoming

Today, we had to kick the father's brother out of a laboring mother's pre-delivery room. He and the patient were having sex while she was 3cm dilated.

The father had gone home at mom's request for her personal pillow and socks.

None of us told the father because that's really not our place. We don't know if he really *is* the father, or if his brother is.

I have two children and can't imagine any woman wanting to have sex while she was in labor.

--Initials and location withheld at request

Better Out Than In

Security was called for a combative patient. The patient was the tallest man I've ever encountered—he must have been almost eight-feet tall, and he was built like a train. When the cops left him in our emergency room, they said he was a semi-professional wrestler. I didn't know if they were joking or not, but it would sure make sense that the man was a wrestler.

We had four male nurses, orderlies, and techs from our department trying to take this guy down, but he was hyped up on drugs and was flicking grown men away like they were flies. It was insane!

Three security guards came down and one guard tasered the patient. It did absolutely nothing to subdue him. I'm not even sure the patient felt it.

One guard jumped on the patient's back, while another one hit the patient in the back of his knees with a baton repeatedly. Finally, the patient started to drop to his knees.

The third guard continued to wrestle with the patient front-to-front, but as he struggled against this Hercules, the guard strained too hard and farted.

I think this really embarrassed the guard because he turned red and gave up on the fight. Luckily, the patient stopped fighting, stared down at the guard, and started laughing his butt off.

Seriously, the only reason the guards were able to subdue that man is because he was doubled over in laughter at our guard passing gas.

The police came back and cuffed the man's arms and legs to the bed. He was later taken to jail.

--P.D.
California

<u>Watch Your Mouth</u>

I work with pediatric patients, so this means I know all the corny jokes and puns there are to be told. I never thought that the jokes I tell children would anger an adult to the point of what happened while I was at work the other day.

It was New Year's Day, and I said to one of my therapy patients, "Man, I remember 2017 like it was yesterday."

I was too busy ribbing with this child to see my coworker—a man I never really talked to because he made it clear he didn't want to interact with coworkers, unless it pertained to the job—come at me from across the room.

He punched me in the back of the head, and my patient, who was in my arms as we were working on walking again, fell. As my patient was sprawled out on the floor, screaming for help, my coworker continued to strike me in my face (and arms, once I managed to shield my face).

My supervisor came in and pulled my attacker off me. My attacker was fired on the spot and the police were called. I was asked if I wanted to press charges, and I answered, "Yes!"

I don't know what's going to happen with this guy, but I hope he gets the harshest punishment possible.

Luckily, my patient didn't sustain any physical injuries, but he was scared half to death.

--Anonymous at request
Wisconsin

Brr, It's Cold Out Here

Where I live, we don't typically get much snow. Occasionally, we'll get an ice storm. I've lived here all my life, and I can count on my hand the number of times we've gotten more than five inches of snow.

Well, I knew it was snowing because all my friends were posting statuses on Facebook. I did not know how much snow was falling, though, because I work in an office building that has no windows. It's perfect for what it's used for: I work every other day to transfer legal hard files to an electronic library.

Before I knew it, my eight-hour-day was up, so I grabbed my purse, put my coat on, and turned off the lights.

When I tried to push the door open, it was stuck. It took about five minutes to get out of the building.

As soon as I stepped outside, the hairs in my nose froze, and I shivered. I almost busted my ass, just from shifting my weight. I looked down. Everything was covered in snow and ice.

Here's the thing: I get in and out of the building by climbing sixteen metal stairs, which are connected to metal platforms (one between the stairs and another in front of my office door). There was no way I would be able to get down those stairs, especially if I was already sliding around when I was barely moving. I may have done slightly better if I had boots on, but I was wearing flats. My feet were numb because I was standing in about six or eight inches of snow.

Not knowing what else to do, I inched to the top of the stairs. I thought I was going to fall twice. I'm about fifteen or twenty feet off the ground on the top platform, so I was extra careful.

Remember when you were a kid, and you sat down on the stairs and scooted your butt down one step at a time?

Yeah, that's how I planned to get down all sixteen stairs.

I can tell you that it's not fun to put your ass in the snow, especially if you were stupid enough to wear leggings and a sweater when the high for the day is 2-degrees.

Oh, man. I was so freaking cold, but I had to get down. I was supposed to play host to my in-laws that night, so I couldn't stay at the office. We didn't even have food or a place to sleep in the office. I had to get home.

On the sixth step down, I thought I was going to be just fine. I thought I could stand, just for a second, to wipe my butt off and try to give myself a pep talk.

As soon as I stood, I slipped, fell down the rest of the first staircase, slid across the platform and under its thin rail, and I landed in the parking lot.

I hit my head on one of those rectangular stone things they put at the front of parking spaces, so you know when to stop.

Thankfully, I was able to speed-dial my husband and simply say, "Work, fell," before I passed out. He called 911.

By the time the paramedics arrived, my body temperature was 93-degrees. In the ER, they brought in some kind of machine to warm me up slowly. The gash in my head stopped bleeding on its own and turned out to be such a small laceration, anyway. The doctor told me I was lucky that I didn't bust my head open, and he didn't know how I *didn't* bust my head open.

I can tell you one thing: I won't be doing that again. I called in and said I won't be returning to work until the snow and ice have gone away. My bosses were okay with that.

--V.F.
South Carolina

I just find it funny how my hospital places visiting restrictions during flu season, telling all these people to stay away if they're showing symptoms of the flu or gastroenteritis, but I can't call off when my temp is 103.4 and I've been on the toilet all day…because there are 'restrictions' involved with the 3,000 hours of PTO time they won't let me use. Just sayin'!

--N.K.B. from Delaware, sounding off on what we're all thinking.

Superior Customer Service

I work two jobs, one of them as an emergency line operator. This call, which was taken a few months ago, was my first call of the shift. I had just gotten done at my first job, and I'd driven straight to the station. This call got me written up.

Me: Thank you for choosing [fast food restaurant]. Order when ready. Er, I'm so sorry. 911, what's your emergency?

Caller: Uh, I think my grandma's having a stroke. She's slurring her speech, and one of her eyes is droopy.

Me: It shows you're calling from 123 ABC Lane. Is that correct?

Caller: Yes. I'm the only one here with her. I've already unlocked the front door. I left it open, so they can find the house and just come in. I have to call my grandpa.

Me: I'd really like you to stay on the line, if possible.

Caller: I really have to call my grandpa, though. Look, I'll call him, and then I'll call you right back. Is that okay?

Me: Yes, that will be okay.

Caller: Okay, give me a minute.

Me: Take your time, and order when ready.

Caller: What the hell is wrong with you? Oh my god. My grandma could be dying, and you keep making jokes.

The caller hung up on me and wouldn't give me a chance to explain when he called back to give me a status update on his grandmother. I felt horrible, embarrassed, and unprofessional. My boss took it easy on me, but the caller and his family complained, so my boss gave me a written warning to satisfy the family's demands for punishment and to 'remind [me] where [I am] in the future.'

Trust me, after that call, I never forgot again.

--J.I.
Oregon

<u>Hereditary</u>

I wish your books were around 10 years ago, because when I was working in the ER, I could have come home with enough stories to give you a few more dozen books.

One thing I remember from my career was this child who'd come in with a condition that could be treated, but not cured. His parents, grandparents, and siblings accompanied him to the ER.

I was in the room as the doctor explained to the family that the child's condition was genetic, and that while the father may not have shown (or ever show) symptoms of the condition, he was a genetic carrier, and therefore, he passed the condition to his child. His parents both suffered from the condition but had no idea it could affect their son or his children.

The patient's parents said they understood everything the doctor was saying, and the grandparents seemed to understand, but it soon became clear that there was still some confusion.

The patient's mother started crying and asked, "Well, if I file for divorce, my boy won't be sick anymore, right?"

"Huh?" the doctor asked, completely lost.

"Well, if it's a family thing," the patient's mother explained, "then I'll just file for divorce and take custody of the kids, and then my boy won't be sick anymore."

This suggestion started a family argument. Finally, the doctor stepped in, told everyone to stop screaming at each other, and explained that the patient would have this condition even if the family separated because genetics didn't care about a marriage certificate or custody agreement.

--G.H.
Washington

I answered a 911 call from an elderly man who was left to babysit his granddaughter, when his daughter was on a business trip. The man was crying because his granddaughter's hair was tangled after a bath, and he didn't know what to do. I calmly instructed him on which detangler I use for my own daughter's hair, and I told him where he could buy a bottle. He sounded so relieved when we ended the call.

--D.E.
Georgia

Can You Hear Me Now?

I worked at a major retail pharmacy. Our building has a drive-thru speaker, which has been convenient for both customers and also staff. However, no system is without its flaws.

I was taking inventory one day, when I thought I heard someone shouting through the speaker. It was a faint yelling, though. As I neared my working area at the window, I could indeed tell that someone was outside, yelling about a medication refill. This woman was screaming that I was incompetent and lazy, and maybe I should do my job and take care of customers.

The problem with this, though, is that there wasn't a car at the speaker.

When I realized the problem, I put on my heavy jacket, braced for the freezing temps, and stepped out through the emergency exit.

"Ma'am!" I called through the falling snow and sleet. "Ma'am! The pharmacy speaker is up there. You're yelling at the film drop-off box."

--D.Y.
Maine

I was taking a shower one night, when I saw a face trying to peer through the frosted glass. I freaked out, and that's an understatement. I screamed bloody murder, tried to hide my naked body by trying to wrap myself in the shower curtain, slipped, and hit my head on the faucet. There was blood everywhere.

My husband had to drive me to the emergency room (where I work), and everyone laughed because I realized about halfway there that the face I'd seen in the glass was my own.

Nobody will let it go. It's been two years.

--A.V.
Kentucky

Uh...

I once had the great displeasure of removing 15 used condoms from a woman's vagina.

She told me the condom package said for the male to take the condom off after use, so she thought that meant she and her partner were supposed to leave them inside of her and the condoms would "I don't know, dissolve or something."

The condoms didn't dissolve. They did, however, contribute to the infection the patient developed.

I will spare you the disgusting details about the condition of the patient's vagina. The infection was quite prominent, I will say that much.

I was professional during extraction, but I left the room and vomited.

I have never met a patient so stupid! That, honestly, has been my most revolting case in nearly 12 years of practicing, and I pray I never encounter anything like it ever again.

On the other hand, I am so glad the patient and her partner were using condoms, but it's only a matter of time before they have a baby, and that scares the shit out of me.

--R.P., O.B.-GYN.
Florida

<u>Freeze!</u>

I took a newly-prescribed medication, and then I realized I was out of toilet paper and milk. I drove down to a retail pharmacy and felt fine as I was walking around.

Well, right after I grabbed the toilet paper, I felt strange, so I dropped the TP in the middle of the store. I felt hot, dizzy, and tired all of the sudden, so I thought I'd go home and sleep it off. Maybe those were normal side effects of the medication. I didn't read the warnings on the prescription bottle, so I didn't really know.

A clerk tried to stop me as I was leaving, but I just waved her off and said, "I'm fine. Don't worry about it."

Out in the parking lot, I kind of felt confused. Now, of course, I realize I shouldn't have been driving at all. I should have called 911. But, at the time, I thought I'd be okay to drive the four blocks home.

I got in my car and was having trouble getting the key in the ignition. Maybe I wasn't lining the key up correctly, I don't know. I just couldn't get the key in, and I was feeling worse with each passing second.

You know, I was so out of it that I never noticed that two police cars pulled up behind me. An officer approached my driver's side door with his weapon drawn, and it scared me half to death.

He ordered me out of the car, and stupid-me was telling him I'd be okay, I just needed to go home.

The officer ordered me out of the car again, and as soon as I got out, I passed out. I hit my forehead on the open car door, and the officer prevented me from hitting my head on the asphalt.

I woke up in the emergency room, with three stitches to close the gash on my head. I was handcuffed to the bed. Those smart nurses realized I was experiencing an allergic reaction (I had just been there the day before for my condition, so they knew the medication I had been prescribed).

It turns out that I never did drop the toilet paper. I thought I did, but I guess I just walked right out the door with it, and that's why the clerk was yelling at me. She called 911 for a shoplifter, and someone else in the store called 911 for an in-process car theft. Nope, the car I was in wasn't my car. I had been so disoriented that I didn't even know I was in someone else's car.

After we all figured out that it was a big misunderstanding, the cops left, and I was placed on a non-critical wing for overnight observation.

Obviously, the nurses told me to never, ever take that medication again.

--U.W.
Indiana

I have been practicing for 26 years and have encountered three patients who've ejaculated during prostate exams.

The last time I encountered this was last week.

My patient panicked out of embarrassment, and he tried to pull away. I'm not sure if it's just the way he pulled or what, but he ran to the corner of the room with my glove hanging out of this bum, and he was crying as he begged me to please leave the exam room.

I complied because I was on the verge of laughing.

--E.C., M.D.
Nevada

<u>Teething</u>

Registration called me up to the front for an urgent situation. When I answered the phone, the registration clerk was so upset that I could barely understand her.

"Calm down," I said. "Take a breath and tell me what's happening."

"This baby," she shrieked. "This baby, I don't think he's breathing. His lips are blue and he's, like, he's not moving."

I smacked a coworker in the shoulder as she continued watching the YouTube video we'd been viewing together, and we both raced to the ER lobby.

The patient's mother was not hysterical, but I wouldn't call her 'calm,' either. Some people have different ways to express emotions, to express panic, so I wasn't judging her reaction to the situation. As soon as she saw two nurses come through the ER doors, she ran to us and handed an eight-month-old to me.

The child's body temperature felt average in my arms. I reached in his mouth with my fingers and shouted back to his mother, "Did he swallow something?"

"I don't know," his mother cried.

I noted a rash around the child's mouth and on his palms and fingers, but I focused on trying to clear his airway.

I flipped the baby over and held him with his chest against my palm and his head cradled in a 'tripod' I made with my fingers. I gave three whacks to his back, hoping to dislodge any foreign body preventing him from breathing.

"Was he eating something before this happened?" my coworker asked, as I called out an order for someone to call a code and get Respiratory down to us stat.

"No," his mother said. "He was just watching TV while I was folding laundry."

"And did you see him with anything in his mouth? Maybe he found food on the floor, or maybe he found something he could have swallowed?"

"I don't know," the woman panicked. "The only thing he had was a tampon."

"A tampon?" asked our doctor, as he was rushing to assist.

The mother nodded. "He's teething, so my friend said to give him a tampon."

To be honest, I don't remember much of the conversation between that moment and what happened a few seconds later. Our doctor slapped at the baby's back and managed to dislodge a slimy piece of cotton that the child had swallowed.

As if things weren't already bad enough, the child had an allergic reaction to the tampon's perfume additive, which resulted in the rash around his face and hands.

The patient and his mother were in the ER for a few more hours, until we were satisfied that we controlled his allergic reaction and that he wasn't going to have complications from the choking incident. We educated his mother on teething practices and urged her not to try giving her child a tampon again. Charge gave the woman a number for our

Infant and Toddler Family Group, and we knew the volunteers there could get her set up with educational literature and vouchers for toys, formula, and health necessities.

--W.J.

Alabama

<u>Whoops</u>

Last week, some woman insulted me as I was working at a fast food drive-thru (I am only a part-time medic, until the station owner approves a new budget). She had no reason to be so rude; I think she was trying to show off for her snooty friends.

Guess who called 911 because she closed her hair in her car door, with her keys locked inside?

This 'lazy loser who will never amount to anything' showed up to jimmy the lock and free her, and then I had to transport her to the hospital because she complained that her head hurt. She wasn't even bruised, just tender from the tension.

She was rude during transport and spent the whole time on her cell phone. She was taking selfies during transport, and at one point, she asked my partner to take her picture because she wanted to send her friends a

picture with her pretending to be unconscious.
I wanted to throw her into the road.

--D.W.
Arkansas

<u>Injustice</u>

I was employed as an RN in the ED for three years. I was used to being hit on by patients, especially when officers brought in subjects for ETOH screens, or when frat boys would come in with injuries that could have been avoided. I always brushed it off.

One night, a guy came in and was flirting nonstop, even after I told him I was married. He didn't care. I treated him, a doctor saw him, and he was discharged. No big deal.

Well, he was waiting in the parking lot for me when I got off work three hours later. That was a big deal.

I immediately walked back inside, notified security, and a guard walked me to my car. I never said a thing to the patient, nor did I look at him. I thought if I ignored him, he'd get the message to leave me alone.

His stalker behavior continued until he broke into my home while my husband was in the shower. Thankfully, my dog (a 55-lb pit bull mix) bit him. My husband heard me screaming, and he (all while wearing only a towel around his waist) managed to subdue the man until the police arrived. The man had to get stitches to his bite wound. My dog was taken by animal control and quarantined for a week, since he was involved in a biting incident. I thought this was unfair, seeing as how the man who stalked me and broke in my house was released and free to do whatever he wanted. He had a trial set for the next month, but he was free to walk the streets until then.

I filed an emergency order of protection against this man, but it was just a piece of paper. I was scared for my life. My husband arranged his work schedule, so he could take me to work and pick me up. I started carrying a knife. We got my dog back from animal control and changed the locks on the back door. I tried to continue with my life, but I didn't want to go to the gym or go grocery shopping. I was afraid the man knew my routine. He had obviously followed me enough to know where I lived.

The night before the man was supposed to appear for his trial, he broke into my house again. This time, my husband wasn't home; he had to fly out of state to attend a business convention.

When the man broke the patio door window, I immediately called 911. I can't explain the helplessness that I felt. Sure, someone knew the man was there, but now this man had 5-10 minutes to murder me, because that's how long it would take for the cops to show up.

I told the 911 operator that the man was reaching through the broken window to unlock the patio door. She told me to hide, preferably in a room with a lock. The only room I have with a lock is the bathroom. I called for my dog, but he was already attacking the intruder, who was now standing in my kitchen, trying to shake my dog from his arm.

I locked myself in the bathroom and told the operator that my dog was biting the man. I asked the operator to please instruct officers to call out to me when they arrived and surrounded the intruder, and I would retrieve my dog. I didn't want anyone to panic and shoot my dog.

Officers came and arrested the man…again. My dog was seized and taken to animal control for quarantine…again.

At trial, the man was sentenced to jail. I awaited my dog's release from quarantine.

Imagine my surprise and frustration to learn the man who'd disrupted my life and unlawfully entered my home not once—but twice—filed a complaint against the city and named me as harboring a 'vicious animal.' What's more is that the city seemed to entertain this man's complaints. I was informed I could not have my dog back, and that my dog was ordered to be euthanized because he had been involved in two biting incidents within two weeks. They cited his breed as support in the decision to euthanize him.

I was beyond a measurable level of anger and stress.

I found that dog behind the gym one night. He was the runt of the litter, and he'd been abandoned. I brought him home and fed him from a bottle for weeks, every two hours. The vet said he couldn't had been more than three or four weeks old. He quickly became my best friend. Admittedly, he grew to act slightly territorial of his home, but the worst act of aggression he displayed was sitting on the couch, growling at the mailman through the window. He was a faithful companion, not just to me but also to my husband. One time, my husband fell off a ladder and hit his head. My dog came to the basement and pawed at me until I went upstairs and could call for help. This dog wasn't vicious. He wasn't a killer. I recognize the potential that any dog has to 'snap,' but I wasn't about to treat my dog like a beast unless I had some indication that he was unstable. I couldn't believe the city wanted to kill my dog for protecting me, for protecting his home.

I protested the city's decision, but they said there was nothing I could do, that the order was final. I found an attorney and we appealed the city's decision. The city tried to tell us that they could euthanize my dog whenever they wanted, and they didn't have to wait for the appeal decision to be made. We had to, basically, get a restraining order for my dog to protect him from being euthanized during the trial.

Volunteers from the shelter—where he'd been housed since the incident—came forward to testify that my dog had displayed 'outstanding' behavior during his confinement. He obeyed commands, passed aggression tests, and he did not fight with other animals during 'exercise time.' I had to plead with a veterinarian from a local university to dispel the rumor that 'once dogs taste blood, they will always crave blood.'

This was a very long, tiresome ordeal. My husband and I exhausted our savings to pay attorney's fees, take time from work, and fit in time for 'dog visitation.'

Luckily, we won our case, and our dog came home. Around this time, I was hit by another whirlwind of information. One of our unit clerks admitted to giving out my personal information to the intruder because she apparently 'didn't like me.' HR stated they couldn't accept testimony from my coworker that stated the unit clerk told her this. Even when the unit clerk admitted this to me and I went to HR, they stated they couldn't do anything about it. I quit my job on the spot, and I don't regret it for one second.

I loosely followed news for the intruder's sentencing. He was sentenced to a minimum-security prison for one year, but was released after three months due to 'overcrowding and good behavior.'

It took more than three months to fight for my dog's life, so it's good to know that our lawmakers don't have a problem letting a dangerous man out on our streets, but they'll be quick to kill a dog for protecting his home.

--Z.W.
Location withheld at request

The most bizarre patient I encountered arrived at the ER via EMS. He was in and out of consciousness and admitted to taking bath salts. He sustained severe burns to his penis and testicles. The patient said he attempted to masturbate with a fresh-out-of-the-oven Cornish hen.

He was flown out to a hospital that specialized in burns, and officers accompanied him because he was violent when he was conscious.

Freaking crazy!

--M.S.
Kansas

We had an alcoholic who was brought in by his mother because he had cellulitis…from injecting alcohol. He said he thought shooting vodka intravenously would help the alcohol enter his system faster. He eventually had to have skin grafts and was in and out of rehabs until he died of an overdose.

--R.A.
New York

Midnight Madness

I was at my in-laws' house for Thanksgiving, and I had to pee in the middle of the night. I sleep in the nude and couldn't find my clothes without waking my very-pregnant wife, so I thought I would risk it. The bathroom was right down the hall, and everyone was asleep, anyway. I could surely get in and out without nobody ever knowing I was up, right?

Well, I hurried down the hall and into the bathroom. The door is misaligned, so you can close it a million times, but it will still pop open. I closed it slightly, and I started to pee.

As I was relieving myself, I heard a loud creak and the door started opening. Scared that my mother-in-law or someone else in the family would see me naked, I jumped. It was purely reflexive.

I was still peeing.

So, not only was I spraying this spotless bathroom with urine at two in the morning, but I also somehow caught my testicles on the corner of the sink vanity, and I felt my skin rip. I looked down, as I was still spraying urine on these hand towels my mother-in-law embroidered by hand, and I realized I was bleeding.

I can't handle blood, so I felt dizzy, and I guess I knocked a picture frame off the wall, which shattered. I remember seeing a big, fat cat push its way into the bathroom. That must have been what opened the door.

I woke up in the ER, with stitches to my foot (I guess I stumbled around and cut my foot on glass from the picture frame as I was passing out). I also had one of those teeny-tiny circular dot Band-Aids on my balls.

My 12-year-old niece heard the commotion and found her naked uncle bleeding and unconscious on the bathroom floor…with my mother-in-law's 18-pound cat sitting on my chest. She called 911 and woke up everyone in the house.

I've never been so embarrassed in my life, and my mother-in-law is still pissed about the towels that I ruined.

--D.H.
Rhode Island

I Saw the Light

Before our station had emergency generators, we were just S.O.L. when the power went out. We kept emergency supplies, such as lanterns and flashlights for when the power would go out, but our group wasn't/isn't the most 'mature' group, so a lot of those lights ended up in bunks so we could read in the dark, used to practice making dirty shadow puppets, and generally carted all over for non-emergencies. This meant, of course, that when we had a real emergent situation, most of the lanterns worked for about two seconds before their batteries went dead, and the rest of the lights, well, we had no idea where they were.

This was the case during a terrible thunderstorm one night. We were in the middle of a tornado warning (that none of us were taking seriously), and we needed those lights.

I found a backpack on the floor and identified it by the stickers on the canvas. It belonged to one of our guys, John, who was out on transport. He was working a 34-hour shift before his vacation time.

"Oh, he has a flashlight in there," someone said.

"How do you know?" I asked.

"He was shining it on a wall, playing with a stray cat, when we were staging last night. He said he always has one in his bag."

We didn't think John would mind if we borrowed his flashlight for an emergency, so I blindly dug through the backpack, until I reached a flashlight on the bottom.

I pressed a switch a few times, but the think didn't light up. I thought the batteries might be loose, so I slapped the thing against my palm a few times. The last time I did that, I heard the flashlight make some kind of whirring noise. I felt around on the thing and something on the end of the flashlight was suctioning my finger.

Right around this time, someone else found a flashlight and shined it on me. I looked down to see what I was holding.

John carried a male sex toy in his backpack. It was shaped like a flashlight, with a 'mouth' where a light would be on a flashlight. I guess it also had a 'blowjob' feature…that I felt when I accidentally stuck my finger in the 'mouth.'

When I realized I was holding John's sex toy, I freaked out and kind of threw the thing 100-feet in the air. It landed on the station couch, where we left it because none of us wanted to touch the thing.

John came back from his run and wasn't even embarrassed that we'd found his toy. He just shrugged his shoulders and said, "I'm here for almost three days, assholes. What'd you expect?" Then he put it back in his backpack and showed us that his *real* flashlight was on his belt.

That was the last time I went through anyone's belongings, so I guess it's safe to say I learned my lesson.

--P.I.
Nebraska

She's a Star!

    I work in an assisted living facility for geriatric residents, and we had an incident I don't think any of us will ever forget.

    Jane was 94 and had no family, except for great-grandchildren, all of whom lived too far away to visit regularly. She didn't let this get to her, though. She enjoyed interacting with other residents' families, and everyone accepted her company with open arms.

    A few times a week, Jane would talk to her great-granddaughter, Joan, on the phone. Joan visited maybe three times a year and always sent Jane care packages. Jane always said that one day, Joan was going to be a famous movie star and move her to California. We entertained this because we wanted Jane to remain happy with life.

    One day, Jane got off the phone with Joan and excitedly called for me. She said that Joan got a role on a TV show and it would be airing that Wednesday, at 10 P.M. She wanted to make a big party of it, by writing out invitations to all the residents and staff. She wanted everyone to attend a 'viewing party' in the commons area, where we have a large television mounted to the wall. She asked if I could bring snacks.

I thought this was a wonderful idea, so I campaigned to my uptight manager for Jane to have this 'party.' What could it hurt? These people deserved to have a little fun, right?

Well, I bought Jane what she called 'fancy' invitations from Hobby Lobby, ordered desserts and finger sandwiches from my friend (she was trying to get her catering business off the ground), and I even got everyone some of those confetti poppers and fun hats to wear. My coworkers helped me decorate the commons with balloons, streamers, and fun centerpieces for the tables. All in all, it was a pretty fun preparation.

It was the big night, and most of our residents were really pushing themselves to stay awake, since it was way past their bedtimes. Everyone was excited. Joan's 'big Hollywood debut' was all anyone had been talking about lately. We were all excited for Jane to see her great-granddaughter on TV.

At 10 P.M. sharp, we turned on the television and punched in the number for some paid movie channel (like HBO or Cinemax). The lineup was off, so we'd missed the opening credits, but Jane wasn't all that worried. She excitedly pointed to the screen and told everyone, "That's her! That's Joan!"

We were all into it, but the staff quickly realized this was a little too, shall we say, dramatic.

It didn't take long to realize—especially when we all watched Jane's great-granddaughter get naked and start having sex with a man—that this was a softcore porn from a series.

I remember very clearly that one of our elderly men said to Jane, "That's a fine-looking girl you have there!"

He said this as Jane's relative was on all-fours, with a man behind her.

Another woman became disgusted and said to Jane, "Your granddaughter is a floozie!"

Jane shrugged off the criticism and announced, "Well, you have to start somewhere, don't you?"

A few residents wanted to go back to their rooms because they were tired, but the woman who complained about Jane's great-granddaughter was the only one who cited that she wouldn't watch 'that filth.' Everyone else seemed highly interested.

We turned off the program, but several residents protested so much that we turned it back on and let them watch.

And that's the night we had a party to let our residents watch pornography in the commons area.

--U.T.
Pennsylvania

I had a patient refuse me as her nurse because she said, "Your name is ungodly."

My name is Dick.

This woman was so upset over my name that she requested another nurse.

She was 70-something, so I doubt I'm the first 'Dick' she encountered.

--D.S.
Maryland

Didn't Think This Through

About ten years ago, I was the nurse assigned to a young gentleman complaining of back pain. During triage, he was noticeably fidgety, and by the time I got him in a treatment room, he added a headache, leg pain, and dental pain to his list of complaints. He wanted narcotics and told me this.

Fortunately for us (but unfortunately for the patient), a hospital in the next county called us and warned that the man had visited that hospital earlier in the day, and he had to be forcefully removed when he was denied drugs.

As soon as the patient learned he would not be getting anything stronger than Motrin, he became belligerent and had us all worried that he would become violent. Our doctor refused to speak with him further, so I was told to discharge him. The patient refused to leave, and I had to threaten to call security or the police, whichever the patient preferred.

He screamed at me, got in my face, and at one point, he flipped the chairs in the room. I couldn't leave the room because he basically had me trapped inside as he threw his tantrum. Luckily, a housekeeper heard the commotion and paged security.

The patient left before security arrived. He broke a window on the way out, and it was clear he had injured himself because there was a trail of blood.

We called the police.

Shortly after the patient left—and before the police arrived—registration hit the panic alarm, which locks down our ER. Nobody can come in, and nobody can leave. Strobe lights flash in the lobby, and the doors leading to the parking lot lock.

What warranted the alarm was this: a gentleman entered the lobby, with a white facial mask on his face. His hand was wrapped in a bloody rag. He was threatening the registration clerks with a gun.

It was clear that it was the patient who'd just left because he was wearing the same clothes and still had his armband on.

About a minute into waving a gun around, the patient started screaming and demanded registration give him a wet towel and call a doctor to help him. He started wiping the facial mask from his face and was crying.

While we were in the back, we could see him running around on camera and screaming, "It burns! Please, get it off!"

Police arrived and placed the man under arrest, but he did have to register for a medical clearance. His hand required sutures, since he cut it breaking the window the first time he left. He was also treated for an allergic reaction. The white paste he smeared on his face to 'hide' himself, as he put it, was Noxzema his girlfriend had purchased and left in his car. He thought we wouldn't be able to tell who he was.

He still didn't get narcotics.

--M.P.
New Jersey

What a Bunch of Crap

    EMS transported a patient to my ED, and I was assigned as his nurse, despite already having five other patients. I was overworked, overwhelmed, and I honestly couldn't handle one more task, but the charge nurse didn't seem to mind.

    When the patient arrived, medics told me to 'have fun,' which we all know is code for 'you're about to hate your life.' The joke was on them, because I already felt that way and couldn't wait for my shift to end.

    Ten more hours of a twelve-hour shift to go. Yay!

    This patient complained of stomach discomfort and fever. I showed the patient where our restrooms were located, explained he could not have food (that he requested within his first five minutes with me) until labs had been completed, and then explained that we were a little backed up, so lab could take a while to come down to draw samples.

When the patient stated he would 'be okay waiting,' I was so relieved. I told him to use the call button if he needed me, try to relax until lab came, and I would be with him as soon as lab gave results to the doctor and me. He seemed okay with this.

I checked with the patient probably every 20 minutes or so. Each time I entered the room, I smelled something foul, but I started thinking maybe it was the patient I smelled. Maybe I just hadn't noticed his odor before. The smell was absolutely nauseating, and I tried to spend as little time as possible in the room. I think lab came down about an hour after the patient arrived, and that's the last time I remember checking on him before his results came back.

When the patient's results came back, we noted he had tested positive for an E. Coli infection, and therefore we began protocol to isolate the patient and transfer him for floor admission. I let the doctor explain this to the patient. The doctor asked me if I had noticed the patient's odor, to which I just nodded and cringed.

Shortly after the patient was transferred upstairs, I went in the room and could still smell something nasty. I had only gone in there to get some tubing from a drawer, so I tried to hold my breath while retrieving the tubing.

'O-M-F-G' was my reaction when I opened the drawer.

The drawer was filled with diarrhea.

I opened the adjacent drawer, and it too was filled with diarrhea.

The patient had filled nine drawers with his excrement, and in the tenth drawer, he left a note on a notepad that had been on the counter. It read, 'I shouldn't have to wait so long for help.'

Never in my LIFE have I been so disgusted by someone's behavior, and I have encountered the 'worst of the worst' of mental health patients and criminals. I have never dealt with someone who did something like that out of spite.

Housekeeping had to come down and remove all the drawers, disinfect them separately, and disinfect the room. We were already seeing triple our normal patient load, so we really couldn't afford to lose a room, but we had to mark it as out of order for the rest of the night.

Housekeeping even had to bring down what they called an 'ozone machine' that they said basically 'put new particles' in the air to diminish the odor. I don't know how that works, exactly, but I know we weren't supposed to go in the room while the machine was running (not that any of us wanted to, anyway).

While I can understand the patient's dissatisfaction with his wait, I cannot understand why he thought it was acceptable to do something so revolting.

--P.D.
West Virginia

<u>Toxic</u>

I used to work on a bariatric rehabilitation unit. We primarily assisted patients with lifestyle changes, and we worked with them to perform basic tasks we take for granted, such as walking from the bed to the bathroom, wiping, or bending over. Our patients were mostly immobile when they entered our unit. Our goal was to never discharge a patient in the same condition in which they were admitted.

One patient, Jane, came to us out of desperation. She stood about 5'5" and weighed more than 600 pounds. She had been bed-ridden for some time; she couldn't roll over, use the restroom on her own, and she had to wear an oxygen mask every few minutes, because even breathing was hard for her. She had multiple health issues and she knew she would die if she didn't do something—and soon.

Jane's adult daughter was to thank for Jane's admission. Jane stated she had always struggled with her weight and body image, but once her husband passed, things 'spiraled out of control.' She later met 'John,' who 'supported [her] in every way.' Jane's weight tumbled out of her control, and when she came to us, she tearfully explained that she wanted to live to see her daughter get married, have children, and see her grandchildren grow up. Jane knew she needed a change.

When Jane first came to us, she was adamant that she had no visitors. She knew the road ahead was a long one, and she said she didn't want anyone to see her in this condition. We respected her wishes and turned her daughter away. When John would call, Jane would ask us to refuse the calls. He sent her letters instead.

A counselor came to Jane's room daily, to assist her in emotional issues. Jane spoke to a nutritionist, and we worked with Jane for months. She lost 175 pounds through a change in diet, water therapy, and daily exercise. She was making wonderful progress and could now walk from her bed to the nurses station, though she still needed a walker.

About six months after Jane had been with us, she said she was ready for visitors. Her daughter came right away, and the two had a long visit.

The next day, I'll never forget, we met John. John was as skinny as a bean pole and arrived with two huge bags of KFC, a bag from McDonald's, one from Burger King, and two grocery bags filled with junk food and soda. He also brought roses.

John was angry when I told him he could not take the food to Jane's room. He threw such a fit that I thought we were going to have to escort him from the floor. Finally, he gave in and asked to go to Jane's room.

I walked John to Jane's room, and I'm not kidding—as soon as he saw her, he frowned and said to her, "Oh no, baby. You've lost so much weight. What happened to you?"

He then went on to belittle Jane for attempting to change her lifestyle, and he must have tried a thousand times to coax her into checking herself out and letting him take her to multiple fast food places and restaurants.

Jane became upset and asked me to make John leave. John didn't protest. Instead, he became irate and said that if Jane wanted to 'ruin' her life, he'd let her. He told her he'd find someone else who appreciated him, and he broke up with her before he left. Jane was sobbing so hard that we had to administer oxygen.

Jane explained to me that she met John on a singles website for 'pleasantly plump' women. She thought John was great because he was kind, charming, and romantic. He always brought her food and gave her everything she wanted. She said that since she'd been in the hospital, she realized every aspect of their relationship revolved around John taking pleasure from watching Jane eat. He'd always encouraged her to gain weight. He wanted her to stay dangerously obese.

Luckily, Jane remained on our floor for several more months, and by the time she left us, she'd lost about half her admission weight, some through exercise and nutrition, and some following a surgery for a lap band. Jane said she was going to live with her daughter for a while, so that she would have someone to help her stay on track in the 'outside world.'

I saw Jane more than three years later, after I had transferred to the OB unit, where her daughter came to give birth. Jane was unrecognizable. She had gone from 600 pounds to maybe 195. She looked happy, healthy, and independent.

I want to encourage everyone out there that change is possible—but you have to want it, and you have to work for it. Don't ever let someone like John convince you that your goals are futile. If you want to change, don't be afraid to ask for help. There are lots of us out there who want to see you do better for yourself.

--C.D.
California

Last year, our hospital saw eight patients who registered with various 'complications' stemming from the anniversary of Michael Jackson's death.

--L.A.
New York

(Author's note: In all fairness, he had some great music.)

<u>Leave That Alone</u>

I am a unit clerk at a busy hospital, and I swear I don't get enough respect at work or out of work. People seem to think that because I'm 'just a clerk' that I'm stupid or something.

I was out fishing with my son, when I saw these two college-aged men using a stick to poke at something in the water. I was trying to mind my own business, but they were being loud and obnoxious, to the point that I considered taking my son to a different part of the park.

"Pick it up," one guy urged the other.

"I don't like snakes," guy B responded. "You pick it up."

"Fine."

I saw guy A lift a knot of snakes from the water, and I called down to them, "You'd better leave those alone. Those are cottonmouths. They can really hurt you."

"You a doctor or something?" guy B snidely shot at me.

"No, but I do work in a hospital, and I've seen those bites before. You guys should really leave them alone."

"Yeah, well," guy A said, "mind your business unless you're a doctor or snake expert."

The men then talked loudly about me and my son, but I just ignored them. Hey, if they wanted to mess with a moccasin nest, that was their problem.

Then, guy B said to guy A, "Go on, pick one up."

My son asked, "Mom, are they really going to try to pick one up?"

I shrugged.

Yes. Yes, they were.

Guy A, who I was labeling the biggest idiot in the world at that time, stuck his hand right in the water, and he lifted a long snake out of the water by its tail.

It took about half a second for the snake to whip its head around and bite the man on his finger. Guy A screamed and dropped the snake, which slithered into the water.

As soon as I saw the blood on guy A's finger, I called 911 without being asked to, and I reported a snake bite. I know I must sound like I'm nosy, but I didn't want this idiot to die right in front of me.

By the time the ambulance had arrived, the man was complaining of chills, was vomiting, his finger was unrecognizable because it was so swollen and discolored, and his friend was panicking.

The next time I was working and saw the medics who transported him, I learned the man was looking at amputation for his finger and grafts of the surrounding area.

He can't say I didn't try to warn him.

--K.D.
Indiana

<u>Wow</u>

I am part of our area's emergency response team. We 'deploy' during natural disasters or when a mass emergency has been declared (an example of this would be a terror attack or a mass shooting). If you have seen the news, you probably have seen footage of wildfires. My team is deployed to treat victims of said fires.

I would like you to know, that despite these people having the ability to—I don't know, open their blinds, and see that the world is up in flames—we still receive just as many calls from stupid and rude people.

For example, I heard a dispatcher ordering a unit to an apartment complex because the caller had a headache for 10 minutes. Another time, as we were waiting for the coroner to make it to our location, we heard dispatch notify our partner unit that they were technically the closest unit to respond to a complaint of 'fingernail pain,' but the operator explained to the caller that all units were busy with the wildfires. The caller apparently 'went off the deep end' and yelled at the operator.

Sadly, I know first-hand that it doesn't matter how bad things are, someone will still call for a non-emergency, and they'll undoubtedly behave as if they deserve to be transported ahead of someone experiencing a life-threatening emergency. This leads me to believe that if we ever experience an apocalypse, you can bet 911 operators and dispatchers will be flooded with complaints of diarrhea and head cold symptoms.

--Initials and location withheld at request

Leave That Alone (Part II)

EMS called in report for a patient they were transporting. They advised us to call the Conservation Department or animal control, and over the radio we could hear people in the background exclaiming they didn't know what to do. Oh boy.

When the patient arrived to the ER, he was crying. This was a 40-something-year-old male, dressed in camouflage and reeking of deer scent, crying hysterically as he was wheeled to a room.

You know, I couldn't blame him.

The patient had a huge snapping turtle clamped to his left hand.

You would think that someone who claimed to be an avid outdoorsman would know not to mess with snappers, but this patient told us, "I knew they bit. I just didn't know they don't let go."

He told us he didn't think the bite would be 'that big a deal,' and he was just 'messing around' with the turtle because he was bored as he was waiting for deer.

Well, none of us knew what to do, either. This turtle was pissed off, and though we tried prying at its jaws, it just wouldn't let go. We asked the unit clerk to call animal control, but their department didn't have anyone on call and nobody would be available until Monday. That didn't help us at all.

I think, at one point, we had everyone from our department either in the room, on the phone trying to contact veterinarians or the Conservation Department, or on the internet, searching for solutions. We were all going crazy, racking our brains to try to get this turtle to release.

In the end, another patient from a few rooms away heard the commotion, and he ended up helping us all out. He suggested we find a 'sturdy, strong stick' and tap lightly on the turtle's beak. This, apparently, would cause the turtle to react with a warning, in which snapping turtles open their mouths menacingly before striking.

It took a few minutes, but it worked. We tapped on the turtle's beak with a toilet brush from housekeeping, and the thing let go of the patient's hand. It kept its mouth open for about two seconds, before it snapped at the toilet brush handle and refused to let go. We moved this 30-pound turtle into a garbage can and waited for someone from the Conservation Department to arrive.

The patient's hand was mangled. We could almost see through his palm from the pressurized 'bite,' and the surrounding flesh was black from bruising. He was immediately transferred to surgery. The turtle was transported to a wooded area near a lake.

I can tell you one thing: you'll never see me messing with one of those turtles!

--A.K.
Ohio

04:00 911 Call

S.U. from Michigan sent in this gem.

Me: 911, what's your emergency?

Caller: I just woke up, and I think I need an ambulance.

Me: What's your medical emergency? Are you experiencing chest pains or shortness of breath?

Caller: No. I had a dream, though.

Me: A dream?

Caller: Yeah. My teeth were falling out. Can you send an ambulance?

Me: Are your teeth falling out now?

Caller: No. They just fell out in my dream.

Me: Are you injured at all right now?

Caller: Not that I can tell, but I think I need to be checked out.

Me: Ma'am, are you aware that 911 is for emergencies only?

Caller: This is an emergency.

Me: How?

Caller: Because dreams can warn you of problems.

Me: Ma'am, I'd say it's safe to say you don't need an ambulance for a dream.

Caller: I want to be checked out. I had a dream that my house caught on fire, and then my aunt's neighbor's house caught on fire. So, I want to be checked out.

Me: For a dream? Even though you're fine?

Caller: I could have a problem. I need you to call an ambulance.

Me: Ma'am, this doesn't sound like an emergency. We like to save our resources for true emergencies.

Caller: *asks for my name*

Me: *gives name*

The caller hung up on me and called the police department to file a report against me. She asked them to arrest me for not doing my job. She eventually got the ambulance she wanted, and I guess they admitted her to the psych floor for mental health issues.

I was in Triage when I heard the registration girl ask a patient, "You stuck what in where?"

That's how you know it's going to be an interesting case.

We sent the guy to surgery because he had a tennis ball stuck in his rectum.

--E.L.
Oregon

<u>Horrible</u>

EMS transported a patient for a complaint of 'feels cold,' and we all thought it was the dumbest complaint ever, especially since it was the beginning of December in Colorado. Like, hello…of course it's cold.

I felt like the world's biggest asshole when the patient arrived, though. She was almost 100 years old and lived alone, with no family to call.

What made me feel worse is that the medics pulled me aside and said they felt I needed to ask one of my nurses to notify Social Services, because the woman's living conditions were horrid.

According to the medics, the woman's rental home did not have running water or heat. The medics found ice formations on the ceiling in her bedroom, where she was found curled under four blankets. She had stuffed old newspapers in her house shoes for insulation, and because she couldn't flush her toilet or bathe, the woman had been relieving herself in a trash bin and washing herself with her Pomeranian's waterless shampoo. The woman finally called 911 because her dog started trembling and she couldn't warm him up.

One of the medics went back to the house and took the dog to his house. Social Services arrived and placed the woman in an assisted living facility that allowed small pets under 25-pounds.

I don't know what happened to the woman's landlord, but I hope he/she was sued and had damages pulled through his/her nose for making an old woman live that way.

--K.W., M.D.
Colorado

I had a guy register for 'excessive gas.' I told him to sit in the waiting room, and someone would be out to get him when it was his turn.

Well, about 20 minutes after he registered, I saw him disappear to the bathroom and stay in there for 10-15 minutes.

He then came to the desk, after cutting in front of maybe five other patients, and announced, "Never mind! It looks like I just had to poop."

We marked him as LWBS, and that was that.

--N.T.
South Carolina

First Time for Everything

I was working my security shift one night, when this car came barreling through the parking lot. It almost took out the back end of a parked car, and the driver scraped the car against the concrete posts we have outside our ER entrance.

I was outside, checking for transients, so I hurried to the car and helped a middle-aged man out of the car and into the lobby. The whole time, he was crying and said that 'something didn't seem right.' He thought he was having a stroke because he was seeing double vision, felt dizzy, and felt sick to his stomach.

A squad car arrived just as I was helping the man to the desk, and an officer approached me right as a team of nurses took the man to the back part of the ER, where they treat patients.

An officer asked me a bunch of questions about the man and told me they received quite a few calls from concerned motorists. They identified the car sitting in the parking lot by the license plate callers had reported, and they wanted to ask the drivers a few questions.

The driver tested positive for alcohol and he was slightly over the legal limit. I was in the back for another combative mental health patient and heard the impaired patient screaming in panic. He said his religion forbade him from drinking and he would never knowingly touch alcohol. He said he was at a party and someone gave him a glass of 'bitter, but good' punch. He had three glasses in an hour's time and when he felt ill, he thought he was having a stroke and made the decision to get on the interstate and drive to the hospital because his insurance only covered 10% of an ambulance transport.

I really felt bad for this guy because he seemed torn up over having alcohol in his system. Not for one second did I doubt his story.

I guess the cop who came in let the guy off with a warning not to drink and drive again, but the guy didn't know at the time that he was drinking, anyway. He said he'd never had alcohol before and didn't realize he was intoxicated.

He asked for a chaplain before he left, but he never really caused any problems for us.

--D.T.
Utah

<u>Arts and Crafts</u>

I work as an RN in the ED, and this moment was my most embarrassing 'mom fail.'

I'm scheduled for night shift and worked the night before, so you can imagine how exhausted I was on Christmas Day, when our family opens gifts at noon. Opening gifts took a good while, and I had to work that night, so as soon as we were finished with opening and playing, I went to bed at 14:00.

My 15-year-old routinely watches my 2-year-old when I'm sleeping. I'm a single mom, and I never mean to make my daughter 'raise' my son, but times are tough, and she is handsomely rewarded for her hard work.

Well, I did get a great sleep. I felt like I'd slept for 22 hours, even though I'd only been asleep about five hours.

I came out of the bedroom to find my daughter feeding my son dinner. I didn't think much of it at first. I made myself some coffee, and then I told my daughter she could go out with her friends, and I'd take over with the feeding.

It took about 10 minutes of feeding my son peas to realize he had a purple bead embedded in his forehead. There was a little bit of blood around it, but otherwise, it was just a bead stuck in his head.

I tried to remove the bead, but he's a toddler and it's almost impossible to do anything with him because he's like an angry octopus.

I couldn't remove the bead, so I went to work and registered him as a patient.

It took three nurses to hold him down and a doctor to remove the bead, *before* he had to get two sutures.

When I asked my daughter about it, she said he had fallen on the floor when she was playing with this jewelry kit I'd bought her, but she said he didn't cry and she never noticed anything different about him. She never gave it a second thought.

I can't tell you how embarrassing it was to have to take my kid in to be seen for something like that.

I called in that night, and everyone's still mad at me for calling in, but oh well.

--D.E.
North Carolina

A thought from the author…

It's truly a sign of times when we have to warn people against eating laundry detergent pods.

Isn't it funny, how we survived through lawn darts, riding in the back of pickup trucks, and riding our bikes down hills without wearing helmets—but these kids who've grown up being banned from playing outside and who know how to work a computer (but don't know how to turn on a vacuum) are growing up eating laundry soap?!

They must have tweaked the soap recipe, because when I was a kid and said a bad word, the last thing I wanted in my mouth was a bar of Irish Springs!

Our patient woke up from anesthesia and started quoting the movie *'13 Going on 30'* word-for-word.

He was a 56-year-old biker in prison for attempted murder.

--K.E.
Wisconsin

Reserved for
Emergencies

I live in the Midwest, and if you've visited or live here, you know the weather is temperamental. Yesterday, it was 70-degrees, and it rained from sun-up to sun-down. Then, overnight, the rain turned to sleet, and what rain had already fallen, froze. This meant the roads were in horrible condition.

Then, around four in the morning, the snow started. By noon, we had nine inches of snow. To some communities, this may not seem like a 'huge deal,' but we are located in a rural community, so while main roads may (emphasis on may, depending on if officials want to go out in the weather) be plowed, most of our roads are not. This is hell on my station and me, because it seems that when weather becomes nasty like this, all of the sudden our runs quadruple. There's just something about bad weather that makes people think it's the perfect time to go to the hospital for something stupid.

It took me more than an hour to get to work, when it normally takes me about 20 minutes. I can't tell you how many run-offs I passed, just because I stopped counting after six. I was going as slow as possible, and my car was still sliding. I have four-wheel-drive, but that didn't help much at all. I saw a semi slide and almost take out another car. That drive was scary.

As soon as I made it to the station, dispatch told me to gear up. I didn't know my first call of the shift would also be my last.

A female called 911 because she said her nose was dry, stuffy, and occasionally bled when she picked it. True story.

My partner and I had to dig our ambulance out of the parking lot before we could go. I fell twice because the parking lot was nothing but a sheet of ice. Shoveling didn't take too long, but it was long enough that my fingers and nose were numb. We cussed a lot, but we eventually made it out of the lot.

We saw two accidents take place within a block of our station. We passed numerous patrol cars, with officers assisting run-off victims. It took us about 10 minutes to get four blocks, and we saw a snow plow go by. The plow was scraping snow off Main Street, but it couldn't make a dent to the ice, so it was pretty pointless for the driver to be out, anyway.

Dispatch notified us that our caller had called again, this time to complain that we were taking too long. Our dispatcher wanted to know our location and expected ETA. My partner had a few choice words for the caller, but dispatch just laughed and said that she'd tell the caller that we were moving as fast as road conditions allowed, and basically, we would get there when we got there.

We were probably going about 15-18 MPH in a 40 MPH zone, when a car slid through an intersection.

My initial reaction was to slam on the brakes. Even though there was a voice screaming in my head *not* to hit the brakes, I did.

Not only did we hit the car, but we also flipped.

The last thing I remember was my partner screaming my name and shaking my arm. My head hurt, and I could feel blood trickling down my ear and onto my face.

Another ambulance was dispatched, and we were transported to the ER. I was mostly unconscious and don't remember much of that. At the hospital, scans determined I did not suffer from a brain bleed, but I did appear to have a nasty concussion. I dislocated my shoulder, cracked two ribs, and I broke my wrist. I have two staples in my head, and they had to shave part of my head because my hair was so thick & in the way. I guess my face bounced off the steering wheel, and I broke one of my teeth. My airbag never deployed, but my partner's airbag worked. He was lucky during the ordeal and only seemed to suffer from mild whiplash.

The driver of the other car was a pregnant woman. She was transported to the hospital, and I could hear her crying while I was being examined. She was in the room next to mine, and I heard her tell the nurse that she worked at a fast food restaurant that wouldn't let her call off due to weather, and she couldn't afford to lose her job. I can't blame her for the crash; anyone could have slid through the intersection. I don't think she or her baby were injured in the crash. I saw her leave when I was being wheeled back from CT.

What I find extremely ridiculous is I learned the woman we were going to pick up called three more times while my partner and I were being transported to the emergency room. She filed a report against the station.

And that's not even all.

I was *still* in the ER when that lady was finally brought in. I heard her screaming because I guess the doctor gave her saline spray and told her to invest in a humidifier. She was screaming at the hospital staff because she said she waited more than an hour to get to the hospital (due to stupid 'ambulance drivers'), and then she was mad because—and this is a real quote— "You assholes take two-minutes to see me and all you can do is tell me to stop picking my boogers."

I was in the emergency room for three hours. I'm typing this to you from my phone, as I'm admitted to a non-critical wing. A surgeon should be here in the morning, to further evaluate my wrist. They're not sure if they're going to have to perform surgery. For the most part, I'm just sore. It could have been a lot worse.

I'm hoping you can share my story because people just don't seem to think before they call 911 during bad weather. I am a person, too. All those medics, police officers, nurses, and doctors are people. We already risk our lives on a daily basis, but to be called to what is clearly not an emergency puts us in dangerous conditions that could be avoided. Am I blaming the caller for our crash? No. That could have occurred during any emergent call. However, this woman's attitude was despicable, and I can't believe someone could be informed that her original medics were involved in an accident, but still not budge on coming to the hospital when it's 2-degrees outside and the world looks like Antarctica.

So, to anyone who gets a little 911-happy when weather is bad, please, please, PLEASE take a moment to ask yourself if this is TRUE emergency. And if it is a true emergency, I guarantee you won't have time to sit around and wonder if it is.

--A.H.

Location withheld at request

<u>Horrible!</u>

I ordered my patient's nurse to administer pain medication, so I was deeply concerned to check on the patient and find him writhing in pain long after the drugs should have kicked in.

The patient stated to me about his nurse, "She said she was giving me Dilaudid. Didn't make me feel better, though."

Two other patients displayed the same levels of pain for their conditions, when they should have been given meds. The same nurse was responsible for administering these medications.

I ordered the nurse to administer medication once more, but this time I kept an eye on the nurse.

I discovered she was pocketing pills and she later admitted to shooting up with a patient's medication, but not before causing a scene and accusing me of harassing her.

I called security and our house supervisor. Law Enforcement was notified. The nurse was fired on the spot, and there's no doubt in my mind she will have her licenses stripped.

While I do recognize that this nurse obviously displayed addiction-like behavior, it's inexcusable to know my patients were being deceived by this nurse and were left to suffer while she stole their medications to get high.

--E.K., M.D.
Virginia

From One Nurse to Another

I have read every book you've written, and I am always bothered by stories of discouraged nurses. Please share my story; if I can help just one fellow nurse, that will be enough for me.

I graduated from nursing school and immediately landed a job on the Critical Care Unit. I had doubts about my intelligence and ability to perform the job, but I shared my doubts with my friends and family, and they assured me I was in the right field for my personality and dedication. I started believing them.

One night, I was ordered to administer a drip. I could have sworn that I checked the dosage and doctor's orders four thousand times, because I was always paranoid about administering an incorrect dosage. I set the drip and throughout the evening, I checked on my patient, who was in stable condition.

Prior to leaving for home, I called the pharmacy to order more medication for my patient, since the drip had run dry. I was informed quite rudely that I needed to double check my information, because there should have been 'more than enough' left for the patient. I was shaking as I pulled the doctor's order. My heart almost exploded when I realized I had set the drip at four times what the doctor ordered.

Thankfully, the patient's health was not affected, but this was still a terrible mistake. This was a mistake that *could* have cost my patient his/her life. I attribute my patient's health to a higher power. Had I made that mistake on the patient down the hall, that patient probably would have died. My patient was extremely lucky that he/she did not expire under my care, all due to this mistake.

I filed a report with the nursing supervisor, had to call my floor supervisor at home, and our legal department was notified. We had to admit the mistake to the patient. I was suspended for two weeks, without pay. I had a date to go in front of the board at my place of employment, and they had to evaluate if I was a danger to patients. I was afraid of losing my license.

During this time, I lost more than twelve pounds, all due to stress-induced diarrhea, vomiting, and loss of appetite. I barely slept. I cried so often and so hard that my eyes were swollen, and my nose was raw. I couldn't believe I had done something so stupid! I told myself a million times that I had no business being a nurse, had no business holding lives in my hands. I was dumb. I was incompetent. I was a danger to these patients. I couldn't be trusted. How could someone as stupid as I graduate from nursing school? How could I have made such an error, especially when I was always afraid of making it?

The board looked extensively at my performance reviews and multiple coworkers testified on my behalf. The hospital believed I had made a mistake, and that I had been punished enough with my unpaid suspension. I would be allowed to come back to work, but I would be supervised for ninety days, during which time I would not administer drugs to any patient without another nurse or doctor present. I was allowed to change bed pans, change dressings, give baths, and assist patients with eating and such. I was not allowed to perform medical procedures, such as administering an IV.

I can't explain to you how humiliated I felt. Most of my coworkers were supportive, but others seemed to be angry that I had become 'useless' to the floor and that their own workloads had doubled because I couldn't help. And they didn't trust me to help, anyway. I told myself that I should just quit. I could try to get a job as a receptionist or maybe go back to school for something else. Then, I realized I couldn't even do that because I couldn't get more student loans to cover another degree.

It took years to move on from that one mistake. I still think about it and shudder. Over the years, I have made more mistakes, just not as severe.

I will tell all my fellow nurses this: You will mess up at one time or another. You will face a question and not know the answer, and then you will feel dumber than a box of rocks because the answer was so painfully obvious. You will doubt yourself. Others will doubt you at some point in your career, whether they choose to show it or not.

I am also here to tell you that you will survive. You are not stupid. You are competent. You are not worthless.

When you are feeling these crippling emotions, stop what you're doing, turn off the world, and breathe. That's right, when you feel like you can't breathe, stop right there, and take a deep breath. Hold it. Let it out. Do it again. Cry, if that's what you need to do. But don't you ever give up. Cut yourself some slack. You are in a field where you go, go, go five to six days a week for ten to fifteen hours a day. You're in a field where some patients only make it out the doors to be wheeled to the morgue. You save lives. You lose lives. You face a million different emotions and sometimes all within the span of an hour. Your brain is crammed with eighteen $300 textbooks worth of information, from how to prepare a patient care chart that nobody ever uses, to what song your brain sings while you perform chest compressions.

During those moments you think you shouldn't be in this field, take a long, hard look at why you chose nursing in the first place. I knew I wanted to be a nurse when I was 12 and my parents took me to see my grandfather after he suffered from a heart attack. We couldn't find his nurse. Everyone else ignored us. I never wanted another family to ever feel that way. So, I worked my butt off to get accepted into the nursing program. And damn, even school was hard! While my friends were at the movies or going to parties or meeting their spouses, I was highlighting pages at a time, learning how to draw blood, practicing what to do during a Code Blue. I loved and hated every minute of it. You know you did, too, but you also know that nothing can ever mimic the feeling we all had when we heard our names with 'Registered Nurse' behind them.

Move on from your mistakes, but never forget them. Learn from what you do wrong. Slow down. Check three times, instead of checking twice. Ask questions. Who cares if that one nurse is snotty to you because 'you should have known that'? Guess what? You know something she doesn't know. And when she started, she didn't know things that her peers knew. It's all part of the process.

So, next time any of you are panicking or feeling discouraged, remember that you are a human being. Remember that we all screw up at one time or another. All that matters about the fall is that you don't stay down. Get up, wipe away those tears, and do the job with all the passion and dedication that you feel in your heart.

--M.P.
Indiana

<u>Lost</u>

Many years ago, before our hospital was rebuilt with an added mental health wing, I received a patient with suicidal ideations. He slit his wrists, but his wife discovered him before he could complete his intentions. A doctor sutured and bandaged his wounds, and I was supposed to keep an eye on him until we could secure transport to another hospital.

I remember quite clearly that I was pulled to a room by a coworker. She needed assistance rolling and cleaning an immobile patient. That took approximately ten minutes.

When I emerged from the room, I went to check on my mental health patient. His curtain was closed, when it had been open minutes prior. I remember feeling angry that his curtain had been closed, just because we had a busybody tech who'd always go by and close curtains, even after we'd asked her not to. I just *knew* she had closed the curtain.

I entered the patient's room, and we both know what we found: definitely not my patient.

Oh boy. I was panicking. I remember facing everyone and shouting, "Hey, has anyone seen my guy?"

Nobody had.

Oh no, no, no.

I scoured our emergency room and lobby, before I finally called for my supervisor and explained the situation. We didn't have security, so we notified the police of a possible patient walk-away. We called switchboard and asked the operator to call a code. It was a discreet code that only hospital staff would understand as a patient missing from a floor. One staffer from each floor was to call the emergency room to hear details of the patient's condition and appearance. The patient was to be returned to the emergency room if he was found on another floor.

We received an ambulance and when EMTs were rolling in, one of them called out, "Hey, someone needs to get to the bay right now!"

Someone else asked why, and the medic responded that there was 'some crazy guy out there, drinking antifreeze.' They couldn't intervene because their own patient was suffering from a heroin overdose.

Three of us raced to the bay and found my patient chugging from a bottle of antifreeze he'd found in the bay. We pleaded with him to come inside, but he wouldn't listen. He only stopped drinking because he stopped to vomit.

I felt horrible about 'losing' my patient. We brought him inside and the doctor ordered a stat-dose of ethanol (I think it was a vodka drip, specifically), following the patient's ingestion of methanol. The patient was eventually transported to a facility that was better equipped for his condition.

I never did get in trouble for that incident, even though I always kind of blamed myself for what happened.

That incident played a large role in the security department the hospital added a few months later. Today, we have strict security measures in place, including badge readers, so only staff members can access certain areas in the facility.

I honestly don't know what happened to the patient, but I hope he got the help he needed.

--M.B.
New Jersey

Lesson Learned the Hard Way

Okay, so I may or may not be a horrible person for 1.) sending you this story and/or 2.) thinking it was so funny.

A new nurse joined our ER, and she was one of those people certain that she knew everything, never needed help, and she also thought she was above everyone—both in her personal life and at work. She acted all high and mighty because she practiced holistic medicine, was vegan, and she taught yoga on weekends. She ordered us around like she was our supervisor. Everyone hated her.

Not only was her attitude atrocious, but she smelled so bad! She didn't have body odor, but she was addicted to these 'holistic' body oils, and she carried what looked to be a small briefcase to work every day. It held a bunch of tiny bottles of oils. She'd rub lavender on her temples for relaxation, rosemary on her forehead for headache relief, and I can't even tell you what else she used because I usually tuned her out as soon as my brain determined she wasn't talking about a patient. I can tell you that some of her oils just flat-out stunk. She wore one oil that she practically bathed in, and I swear to you, she smelled like bacon bits—you know, those hard crunchy 'bacon' pieces you sprinkle on salads.

Well, one night, this nurse was complaining loudly that a patient 'smelled disgusting.' We had to pull her aside and scold her. The patient was a 92-year-old woman with dementia. She couldn't control her bowels or bladder. This patient was dying, and I mean literally. She was transferred from the hospice floor because they weren't sure what was causing the patient to have seizures, and they didn't want her to suffer. Our nurse was being so loud as she complained that we feared the patient's family would hear. The nurse didn't think any of this was her fault, and she said that she couldn't work under those conditions, especially when she forgot her oils at home.

Well, we didn't care if this nurse had to suffer or not. We *did* care that we were going to have to spend the next 10 hours with her, and if she didn't stop bitching about everything, one of us would be going to jail for strangling her. Someone suggested to the nurse that she rub Vicks under her nose and wear a surgical mask in attempt to mask the odor. She refused to do this.

Finally, someone else told the nurse she could order peppermint oil from the pharmacy, and it could be tubed to us.

In case you've never worked with peppermint oil in a hospital setting, it's not quite like the oils our nurse used. She didn't know that, though.

None of us stopped her as she dabbed this stuff on her temples in large quantities. She even put some under her nose.

It took maybe 30 seconds until her eyes were running so much that she couldn't see, and she was coughing from how strong the smell was. She tried to go to the bathroom to rinse the stuff off, but she ran into a door and some of us were laughing so hard that we were crying.

Again, I'm probably going to hell for thinking that was hilarious, but I can tell you this woman was so nasty to everyone that she deserved every last bit of that moment. She was eventually fired because nearly every patient she treated reported her, which drew concerns from HR.

--T.R.

Texas

OB nurse here.

A few months ago, we received an admit who was experiencing active labor.

She asked everyone she encountered, "How long will this take?"

She wanted to pop out the baby, so that she could go home and watch a movie because, "I only rented it for one night and don't want to have to pay a late fee."

We all told her it would take as long as the baby needed to come out, which turned out to be about 14 hours in her case.

--P.H.
Utah

I introduced myself to a patient from an SNF. She clapped excitedly and said to me, "My goodness! You look just like that young rapper that my son likes so much. You know, Nelly!"

Kerry, I am a 37-year-old white-as-white-can-be male who's going bald.

Maybe she was thinking of another rapper, I don't know.

All the nurses thought it was hilarious. I'm still confused.

--T.W., M.D.
Michigan

<u>Oh, Baby</u>

OB staff members have sounded off loud and clear. Here are a few things they deal with on the baby wing:

It's more common than you'd think, when new mothers and fathers immediately ask me, "How much does [the baby] weigh? How long is he/she?"

Well, I'll be happy to tell you, if you give me more than two seconds of the baby being on the outside world.

Someone should invent implants that turn your arms into a scale and measuring tape.

--D.S., O.B.-GYN.
Washington

I've been on my unit for five years and have been asked three times, "Is he circumcised?"

Um, well…You're asking me that while you're looking at an ultrasound, so…

--R.A.
Florida

One time, I had a father literally push me out of the way, so he could continue taking pictures of his new son.

All the pictures he was taking were of his son's genitals.

Dad was sending pictures of his kid's genitals and then calling his friends and family, so he could brag about his son's 'endowment.'

--M.L.
Maine

I can't tell you the number of new parents who see their babies' 'cone heads' for the first time and completely panic.

One dad threatened to walk out on his girlfriend, stating, "I can't handle a kid with a deformity."

We had to sit dad down and explain that the child's head would eventually 'go back' to a 'normal' shape.

--S.T.
Rhode Island

One time, I was checking vitals on a woman in active labor. She grabbed my arm and explained that she wasn't sure if the baby was her husband's or her boyfriend's. She explained that, if the baby's father was her boyfriend, there would be a 'really big problem' because her boyfriend was black, while she and her husband were white.

I'm not even kidding...This woman knew her husband would miss the birth because he was on military business, so she asked, if the baby was born black, if we could lighten his skin, "you know, like they did for Michael Jackson?"

The woman gave birth to a snow-white child with blue eyes and blonde hair. Her husband showed up two days later, and nobody ever said a word, though my coworkers said the woman asked them the same thing.

--T.Y.
California

We kicked out a new mom's sister, at request of the family.

The sister arrived at the hospital drunk, and then she made a comment about how the baby's 'thick' lips would be useful in performing blowjobs when the child grew up.

We had to call security because the woman was belligerent and then puked in the waiting room.

--O.M.
Nebraska

"Ugh, she's so wrinkly! How am I supposed to take good pictures, if she looks like a prune? Just put her over there or something, until she's not wrinkly."

Real quote from a mom who spent an hour following birth crying because her baby 'wasn't as cute' as she thought she'd be.

Wow.

--D.U.

North Carolina

I called DCFS after hearing mom tell her obviously-tweaking husband, "Man, I can't wait to shoot up."

She seriously called her dealer and he brought drugs to the patient's room.

Her baby was two-hours old.

The dealer was arrested on site, and DCFS took temporary custody of the newborn.

--T.E., O.B.-GYN.

Illinois

I work at a high-traffic inner-city hospital, and while the scenario has become somewhat of an urban legend, I can verify we *do* see several patients per year, who present with cell phones stuck in their rectums. Most of them have had to go to surgery to have the phones removed, but a few have been lucky enough that our staff could dislodge the devices in the ES.

Please, for the love of God, don't stick anything up there unless you're prepared to explain it to the ES staff.

--L.W.
New York

Gotta Believe in Something, Right?

My patient, Jane, presented to our local emergency room with complaints of dizziness and shortness of breath. She was immediately sent to my office for a referral.

Jane appeared to be a healthy woman in her mid-30s. She abstained from drinking, and she'd stated she had never smoked tobacco. It was with deep regret that I had to inform Jane that the spot discovered by emergency services staff was non-small cell cancer, and it was at Stage III.

I discussed options with Jane, as well as 'estimated' recovery rates and/or chances of remission. I spoke of chemotherapy and even holistic options (I do not agree with these methods and made that clear, but I always try to explain every option to my patients). Jane was quiet, which is not an unusual response for someone in her position.

As I was showing Jane an illustration and explaining a surgical procedure, Jane blurted out that she wanted to refuse treatment. This is not unusual, either. Over the years, many of my patients have refused treatment, usually based on their religious beliefs or their overall 'closure' with life. I respect my patients' wishes.

When Jane mentioned a 'higher power,' I assumed she meant God. I have many religious resources to offer; several churches in our area provide group therapy for cancer patients, and I have these meetings organized by denomination.

I asked Jane, "Would you like a number for someone at the church?"

She appeared puzzled and stated, "No. I'm an Atheist."

Okay. Maybe she believed in another power, such as the power of the Earth or something else. I've met patients with nearly every kind of belief that you could imagine.

It took a few minutes to understand, but Jane finally said she believed in an extraterrestrial savior. She stated that she did not believe in religion or creationism stories that many have come to know and trust. Instead, she believed that an alien species had genetically engineered human beings as 'tests,' and that if she had cancer, she was 'absolutely positive' that this alien lifeform would 'either cure or mark [her] as a failed experiment.'

I didn't know what to do or say. I wanted to ask Jane if she would possibly arrange a mental health evaluation, but I think she realized that I was thinking, 'WOW.'

She assured me that she realized her beliefs were against what society would consider 'normal,' but that was her faith and asked me to respect it.

I was able to convince Jane to return for monthly checkups, and she returned faithfully for three years (refusing all treatments and/or medications), before the cancer ended her life. Not once did she stray from her beliefs in extraterrestrials.

--J.D.H., M.D.
Arizona during story's timeframe

Party On

My hospital is near a popular vacationing spot for celebrities, and boy, we have seen our share of movie stars, singers, and models. I'd say we've seen a mix of down-to-earth and 'someone needs to knock you off your high horse; come over here and let me do it for you' patients. High-profile celebrities, you know, the 'best of the best' are usually the 'worst of the worst,' just because I think they've let stardom go to their heads, and if we do interact with them, they're rude as all get-out. Like, chill. I'm not collecting your blood to sell it on eBay; your doctor just wants to know how much alcohol you've had with your cocaine.

One year, we received a patient who is/was well known, but not particularly active anymore. He was nice to staff, but he was excessively flirtatious and somewhat cocky. I was his nurse.

First off, while this patient maintained in interviews and to fans that he practiced sobriety, he was loaded when he arrived in our department. I had to ask him our usual triage questions, and while he was in the bed in his costly private room, he told the truth. To my inquiry of whether he used alcohol and drugs, he replied, "Yeah, everything you've heard of and shit you've never heard of."

He clicked his tongue at me and said with a laugh, "I can tell you that because you can't tell all these people I lie to."

When I asked the patient why he lied to the media and his fans, he gave me an answer I respected. He said, "Because that shit will ruin your life. Nobody needs to go out and do all this shit, just because they see me doing it and think it's cool. It's not cool to nod out and wake up in your own piss and puke, and not know where the [eff] you are, with three women you don't know who could be dead on your floor from an OD. I should be dead by now."

The patient's answer to if he was sexually active was, "Yeah. At least twice a day."

I can't say I was all that shocked to see the patient in the department. Decades ago, he was known for sex, drugs, and rock & roll 24/7. I guess sometimes you don't grow out of that behavior.

The patient admitted to being 'drunk off [his] ass' and trying to climb lattice work so he could sit on his roof and 'roll a joint and eat a taco.'

He didn't seem upset in the slightest about his multiple fractures and learning he'd have to go to surgery, but he expressed multiple times that he was 'bummed' about losing his weed and smashing his taco.

For the record, when word got around that he was hospitalized, none of the reports told the truth. The announcement from his publicist basically gave some 'it was just a common accident' claim and stated the patient had been sober at the time.

My official statement on that was: "LOL, bullshit!"

That man was probably my favorite celebrity to interact with because he was so brutally honest about his addiction and reasoning behind keeping it out of the news.

He grabbed my butt a few times, but he was funny and ended up apologizing, so I didn't hold a grudge. I can at least say a famous person thought I was cute.

--Initials and location withheld at request

(Author's Note: This story was edited prior to submission and edited slightly by me prior to release. Details have been omitted and/or altered, so that the patient's privacy cannot be compromised.)

<u>Uh, Oops</u>

My patient was a college-aged female with the complaint of a 'lost tampon' in her vaginal cavity.

This patient was rude and came to the ED with about 20 of her friends, and that number is not an exaggeration. If anything, I may have undercounted how many peers she brought for 'support.'

We had our first trouble with this patient before she even registered, because all 20-something of her friends wanted to pester security, registration, and other patients. She was registered and sent to the waiting room. She and her friends threw a fit about this, and some of her friends were escorted off the property by our security department. The patient and the rest of her friends then went to the waiting room and 'took over' the room, by demanding ill patients and families 'get the hell up,' just so the female and her friends could sit where they wanted. It didn't matter that half the waiting room was empty; these girls did this because they were bitches, pure and simple.

I had heard everyone complaining about this patient, so I wasn't thrilled when charge told me she would be my patient. *Sad face.*

When I called the patient, she and all her friends came to my triage room door.

"Who's the patient?" I asked.

The woman stepped forward.

"We do not usually allow anyone else in the room for vaginal exams, unless they're family members," I said. However, since I didn't want any trouble or big ruckus, I said to the patient, "But if you want to pick one friend to come with you, that will be okay for this visit."

Of course, this caused an uproar because the patient and her friends started screaming at me that they could do what they wanted, when they wanted, and I had no right to tell the patient how many people could be in her room. And dear freaking lord, the list of what they were screaming about just goes on and on and on and on.

Security had to get involved (again), and the patient's entourage dipped (again), so I won that fight and only one friend came back to the triage area. The patient and this friend weren't happy, but oh well.

Triaging this woman was a nightmare in itself. She didn't want to answer any questions. She kept asking what they had to do with anything, and then she flat-out told me that some of the answers were none of my business. I tried to explain that every question was pertinent to offering the best medical care we could provide, but she was rude. I marked most of the questions as 'PT REFUSED.'

I escorted the patient and her friend to a private exam room and gave the patient a gown. I instructed her to disrobe and put on the gown while I was gone to get paperwork and supplies. She argued about this, too. She was disgusted by—get this—the color and the fabric of the gown. She demanded that I get her a plush robe, and she stated she wasn't going to wear the gown.

Okay, whatever, I wasn't about to argue with the girl. I said, "If you want me to examine you, you'll be on that bed and nude from the waist-down by the time I return."

The girl, I swear to God, she said to me, "I could tell them you tried to rape me, and then you'd be in jail."

You know what happens when you say things like that? You get a nurse who returns to the room with the charge nurse, house supervisor, and a patient advocate as witnesses.

The patient was pissed about having 'so many people' in the room, and she denied ever have said the rape-thing to me. My coworkers know me well enough to know I would never lie about something like that. The patient wasn't my 'type,' anyway, because I have a thing for males, if you catch my drift.

The charge nurse insisted upon remaining in the room and told the patient she was there to 'monitor my technique.' The patient and her friend complained, but again, oh well.

We had to get on the patient's friend for trying to use her cell phone to record the procedure (while standing behind me). We don't allow pictures or video-recording in our department, and we especially do not condone patients' friends and families taking cell-phone recordings of vaginal exams, with the patient's genitals in full-view. We threatened to remove the patient's friend from the emergency room, so she literally stomped her foot and went to the corner. She said, "I'm live-tweeting everything you guys are saying and doing. Expect a lawsuit."

Ohhhhhhh myyyyy gooooooosh.

Well, I was 'digging around' the patient's vaginal cavity with my fingers and couldn't seem to feel a rogue tampon. I couldn't see anything with my naked eye and pushed my hands in a bit further, while stating I may have to call the doctor in the room.

You know what the patient did, while my hand was still in her? She sat up and said with a laugh, "Oh my God, I didn't put a new tampon in."

"What?" I exclaimed.

"I remember. I was only spotting, so I didn't put a tampon in. Then, it got bad, so I went to take the last tampon out, but I just remember that I never put one in."

Really? You *suddenly* remember this, with my fingers halfway to Beijing and covered in blood? We really went through all that, just for you to suddenly recall you didn't even put a tampon in?

I didn't sigh or anything as I removed my gloves and continued washing my hands, but the patient accused me of 'having a shitty attitude' when I told her that I would send a registration clerk in to verify her insurance and contact information. The patient then went on to inform me that she 'wasn't paying for shit' because she didn't have a problem, so our hospital 'couldn't' bill her.

By this point, I think even charge wanted to ask the girl, "Have you ever been punched in a throat by a licensed professional?"

Neither of us said that, of course.

One of the registration clerks left the room and gave a light grunty 'scream' as she slammed the patient's forms in front of me. She said, "I hate that patient."

I just nodded in agreement but couldn't say anything because I was afraid I'd go off on a long rant.

"She said she was going to sue me for illegally collecting her information," the clerk said. "And then, she refused to give me insurance information. I found it in the system from [another hospital] and told that girl that it was too late, that I found it. And then she told me I couldn't do that, that it was illegal, and she was going to file a complaint."

This clerk was worried because her boss scours charts for billing mistakes and often blames the clerks if a patient refuses to answer billing questions. I've seen this firsthand and think it's ridiculous, because sometimes you have patients who are assholes and go through life like they were put on this earth to make everyone's lives miserable.

When I went to discharge the patient, she demanded that I give her free meal vouchers, taxi vouchers, and 'free gifts.' The gifts she was referencing were hospital socks, towels, blankets, and pillows. I point-blank told the patient I wasn't giving her anything but a packet of papers explaining the procedure performed and an after-care plan.

I was called in by HR the following business day because the girl wrote a scathing email to our CEO and accused me of inappropriate behavior. She also complained about the registration clerk. She threatened to file a lawsuit against the hospital. Luckily, my boss was in the room with me, and I documented the patient's threatening behavior and HR received multiple confirmations of the patient's behavior from registration and security.

And, you know what? I hope her parents' insurance company bills that girl for every single penny they can get for wasting everyone's time and being such a pain in the ass.

--T.O.
Indiana

Our department has seen an unusual number of 'wax fruit' cases over the years.

I have been on shift for a wax banana vaginal injury, wax grapes stuck in a man's rectum, and know of at least three other cases where wax fruits have been used in sexual escapades gone wrong or have been used as weapons during domestic altercations.

--A.L.
Wyoming

<u>Where's My Money?</u>

I won't lie. I borrowed money from my friend, and then we got in a fight over my (now-ex) girlfriend. My ex was cheating with my friend, so when I ended my friendship, I honestly thought, 'Screw him and his $80.'

Well, 'John' wasn't about to let that $80 go. Due to him sleeping with my girlfriend and me moving out, I was broke. By broke, I mean I was eating nothing but Ramen, was behind on bills that were in my name from living with that succubus, and all my savings went toward renting another house and setting up utilities there. I didn't know when I'd have the cash to pay John. It really wasn't something I even cared about until…

John showed up in the ER one night.

I work in the ER as an orderly/CNA. If I don't have patients to transport from/care for in the emergency room, I am supposed to go to other floors and assist, so it's not like I have a lot of time to sit around and diddle at work.

I told John to leave, and I told him I'd pay him *after* I took care of my own financial situation. He was mad and tried to fight me, but a nurse called security and John was sent home.

John started registering as a patient, just because he knew I was responsible for escorting patients to ancillary departments and to the restroom, if they needed assistance. John was an able-bodied jock, but when he registered as a patient, he 'suddenly' couldn't walk to the bathroom on his own. He also came in for what doctors suspected to be self-inflicted head injuries, just so he could ask to go to X-Ray. I had to escort him around the hospital, and the whole time he pestered me about money.

I think John registered four times before a coworker gave me the $80 to pay John…I think each of his ER visits were $800, minimum. Yep, he wasted time and resources, as well as ran up around what I'm estimating to be $5,000—just to get his $80.

--M.W.
California

<u>Difficult Choices</u>

I worked in a busy inner-city ER for many years, and one year, a woman named Jane became one of our 'repeat customers.'

At first, Jane would come in for minor injuries, such as finger sprains or she rolled her ankle.

Soon, Jane's injuries were much more serious. Some nights, she'd come in with lacerations to her body and bruises to her face. We suspected she was involved in an abusive relationship, but she never wanted to talk about her injuries. Sometimes, she wouldn't even stay for treatment; we'd get her checked in and she'd be gone by the time a doctor went in to see her.

Several of the nurses slipped Jane business cards for various women's shelters and domestic violence organizations. Still, Jane kept seeing us.

One night, I had been trying to dismantle an old brass daybed from my spare bedroom. I pulled and pulled at one of the bars, until—surprise!—it flew up and hit me in the nose. I was stunned for close to a minute and my nose was bleeding. I was disappointed to see that I also had a black eye. And I had to go to work that night.

Everyone asked me if I had gotten beaten up. It started as a joke, but then it became annoying. I couldn't seem to catch a break. I sneaked outside to smoke, and lo and behold, there was Jane. She was crying and was still wearing an armband. I guess she had checked in before I had arrived at work and left before I ever knew she was there.

Jane asked if she could bum a cigarette from me, so I gave her one. I noticed her lip was busted open, and she had faded abrasions mixed with fresh ones.

She motioned to my face and asked, "Your boyfriend hits you, too?"

I frowned and shook my head. "I hit myself in the face with a brass pole."

"Now, that's an excuse I've never used," Jane said with a weak laugh.

Within hospital policies, I probably should have never said anything, but damn, I'm so glad I did. I lost my temper with Jane and demanded, "Why don't you ever reach out for help? You keep coming in here, over and over, but how many more times will that happen, before you're brought to the morgue instead of to the ER?"

Jane started sobbing and I felt terrible. I almost threw my half-smoked cigarette on the ground and went inside, but I decided I was going to stay and smoke because I didn't know when I'd have another chance. We stood in silence for a few minutes.

As I was turning to go back in, Jane said quietly, "None of the shelters take dogs."

"Huh?" I asked.

"My dogs are nine and eleven," she cried. "No shelter will let me go because I have dogs. But they're going to die soon, so if I just keep my mouth shut and stay, I can be with them."

She went on to explain that her parents had purchased the dogs as puppies. When Jane's parents died, she took the dogs. They had been 2-years and only a few months when

Jane had taken them in. She had lived alone for a long time and met 'the one.' Her relationship started off as a match made in heaven. They discussed marriage and he asked her to quit her job and stay home. He gradually became more controlling and more abusive. Jane didn't have a job or a place to go.

I told Jane to come inside, that I would call a few shelters and speak with the administration. She told me no, that she had to go home before her boyfriend woke up and realized she was gone.

With a dry laugh, Jane said, "Don't worry. You know I'll be back."

I was so worried about Jane for three days. I had called all over the city and, sure enough, none of the shelters allowed residents to have pets. I tried to explain the situation, but nobody seemed to care. They were strict on their policies, they said. They had rules for a reason, they said.

Jane came in again, and this time she was in the worst condition I'd ever seen her in. Her nose was broken, she was missing teeth, her earlobe had been ripped from an earring being snatched from her ear, she was missing patches of hair, she had cracked ribs, and she was so bruised that she cried when we had to move her. She had been brought in by a Good Samaritan, who'd found her crawling down the alley behind her house. Her boyfriend had abused her and locked her out. He had discovered that she had reached out to a shelter and was giving her a 'warning' to never do it again.

Everyone knew Jane needed to get out of that house and there was no time to argue, especially since we were notifying law enforcement. I'm going to be honest here and tell you that I did some illegal things that would—not could—would have cost me my job. They were all worth it.

Jane had just gotten the orders to be admitted upstairs when I went to visit in her ER room. I told her I wanted to foster her dogs until she could get back on her feet. We didn't know how else we could get the dogs out of the house without her going back for them, so she told me when her boyfriend went to work, told me what kind of car to look for in the driveway, and then where to find a spare key.

So, I maybe broke a few laws and policies, and I was scared out of my mind the whole time, but I claimed I was sick, left work early, and drove over to where Jane was living. I found the spare key and entered the house. Jane's two very-fat Basset Hounds never even barked at me. I don't know if it was that they smelled my dog, or if they were just old, or maybe it was a mix. They didn't look like they could do much harm, anyway; they could hardly walk faster than a snail can scoot.

I loaded up the dogs, locked up, and I high-tailed it out of there. Jane didn't care what happened to her clothes. Her boyfriend had destroyed all her family heirlooms that she had when she'd moved in with him. She didn't have anything worth taking (her words), except for the dogs.

The next morning, I called to talk to Jane, but she had been placed in a shelter. She left me a sealed envelope with her caseworker's name and phone number. I contacted her shelter caseworker and after some time (and jumping through hoops to prove that I would be no harm to Jane and had no connection whatsoever to Jane's ex), I finally was able to communicate to Jane that her dogs were safe. They had instantly become part of the furniture and rarely did anything else besides sleep or eat. My young dog tried to play with the duo, but they kind of rolled their eyes and sighed until my dog gave up and brought his toy to me instead.

I fostered Jane's dogs for four months, until she saved enough money from her new job to find a pet-friendly apartment. During those months, we met at a park or at various public places, and she would have 'visitation' with her pets.

Jane and I are still friends. Her dogs passed away some time ago, and she eventually adopted a new dog. We have doggy playdates. Jane went back to college and has a nice job, and she has recently purchased her own home.

I left my ER job so I could get accredited to work in a women's outreach shelter. We offer counseling services, relocation assistance, and legal services. I loved my ER job, but I find this job much more fulfilling.

Since I've been doing this job, I can't tell you how many women confess that they 'can't' leave because children or pets are involved. I want to tell everyone this: there is hope. Don't ever lose sight of hope. Please reach out if you need help. More people are willing to help than you realize. You deserve so much more out of life than staying with an abusive partner.

Jane has asked that we keep our location and any identifying information private.

(Author's Note: If you are in an abusive situation, help is available. Call The National Domestic Violence Hotline at 1-800-799-7233 or
1-800-787-3224 (TTY for Deaf/hard of hearing))

<u>Don't Worry!</u>

I'm a nurse at a maximum-security corrections facility. Patients come to the infirmary for initial check-ups. I usually handle cases of stomach ailments and such. Every now and then, we'll see fight victims come through, or we'll have a patient we need to transport to the hospital. My job is fairly easy.

One day, I was distributing medications to inmates and noticed one patient had been written a prescription for antibiotics. These pills looked like they were made for horses.

I handed one inmate a small plastic cup, which was filled with two pills, and I said, "They're on the large side, so if you have trouble swallowing them, we can probably get them crushed up and put in applesauce for you."

I kid you not, the inmate looked me square in the eyes and replied, "Don't you worry, I used to swallow rubbers filled with heroin. I think I can handle some medicine."

I didn't know how to respond, so I kind of just blankly stared at him.

Well, okay.

--M.R.

Mississippi

<u>For Real?</u>

I registered this college girl once, and it took forever and a day to do anything because she wouldn't stop crying. I could hardly understand anything she said, and by how worked up she was, I thought she had been assaulted or something.

This girl was so hysterical that I finally gave up on registering her properly and entered her as a Jane Doe with condition unknown. When you do that around here, rest assured several nurses will come up to your desk or call, just to know why you entered a patient that way.

"She's hysterical," I explained to the unit clerk, who was relaying my responses to the charge nurse.

I heard the charge ask the clerk a question, to which the unit clerk asked me, "You couldn't get her name or anything?"

"No," I said. "She's really upset."

"No," repeated the unit clerk. "The patient is upset."

I started laughing because I found it hilarious that the unit clerk was forced to act as a messenger, and we were basically playing the game 'Telephone' while we were on the phone. I still don't know why the charge nurse didn't just call me herself.

I heard the charge nurse complain some, but then she came up to the front. The crying patient was sitting on a bench by the door.

"Honey," charge asked the girl, "what's wrong?"

The girl started sobbing all over again. Her face was red, and she had snot dripping down her face. It was gross.

After 10 minutes or so, the girl finally calmed down and said, "I started seeing this guy, and we had sex."

Oh boy. I knew where this was going. The girl was about to tell us that she found out her boyfriend was cheating, so she needed an STD test, or maybe she wasn't on birth control and needed a pregnancy test.

"And I just found out he's allergic to peanuts!" the girl exclaimed.

The charge nurse shot me a look that said, 'I really don't freaking know,' and I returned the look.

"What has you so upset?" the nurse asked.

The patient cried so hard that she almost vomited, but she finally screamed, "He didn't tell me before we had sex! He just gave me his allergy! I freaking love peanut butter, everyone knows that!"

The charge nurse started laughing because she thought the girl was joking, but we quickly learned the girl was being serious. It took the charge nurse about ten minutes to convince the girl that she could not contract allergies via sexual contact.

--N.L.
Missouri

What's Your Emergency?

My report went as follows:

"PT dispatched 911 @ 02:00 because god-freaking-forbid they have to drive themselves to CVS in a snowstorm. They'd rather risk my life to get their Vicodin and Oxy scripts filled. PT smelled of bologna and ETOH, which begged me to almost ask, "What do you do with your life?" PT behaved erratically and rudely during transport, which warranted treatment of slap across face, but I withheld. PT then demanded I take them to Taco Bell, even though I haven't eaten in 13 hours because people keep calling 911 like we're chauffeurs."

Delete, delete, delete

"PT dispatched 911 for transport to CVS to pick up prescription."

--F.R.
Ohio

Besides rare instances when persons with disabilities/LOC/elderly/extreme instances, we at the ER are **NOT** responsible for finding you a ride home!

No, it is *not my job* to drive you home.

No, I *can't* give you money for a taxi.

No, I *won't* call 911 back to take you home.

No, I *don't have free bus passes.*

It is YOUR responsibility to get home.

Say it again for the people in the lobby. They didn't hear you the first time because they were too busy complaining and threatening staff.

Um, How 'Bout No?

Nurses, doctors, EMS, registration, and even firefighters have sent in some ridiculous patient requests. Here are a few:

I work on ICU and had a patient who'd already been admitted for four days. He had been a pain in everyone's backsides from the moment he was on our floor.

This man rang his call bell constantly to request specific foods (03:00 and he wants me to call the cafeteria for pudding), asked us if we could contact our hospital's cable provider to add channels to the lineup, and one day he literally called us every 15 minutes, demanding that we open/shut his blinds, because the sun kept moving into his eyes, but he wanted sunlight in his room.

We were fed up. I understood he was probably going stir crazy, but we had other patients, and we were short-staffed.

The final straw for me was when the patient hit his call light and demanded that I give him a massage. He said it was my job to make sure he was comfortable, and if I declined, he would rate his stay the lowest possible.

I told him no, that I would *not* give him a massage.

Yes, he did mark his patient care survey with all bad reviews.

Our Director made a special trip to the floor to 'observe' how we interacted with patients, all due to one man's revenge-review.

It wouldn't have been so bad, had the Director not told us that from then on, "What the patient wants, the patient gets."

Our administration cared more about sucking up to patients to continue getting great marks, which in turn would lead to funding (when none of us were getting raises), than he cared about hospital staff.

I stayed with the hospital for two more months, but in that time, we lost four nurses and a doctor even resigned.

Sorry, but sometimes saying 'no' to the patient is what the facility *really* needs.

--K.S.

Missouri

My patient was between the ages of twelve and fifteen. He was immobile and non-verbal, following a terrible accident. His parents paid for in-home care, but not full time. I would visit his home daily, usually for about two to three hours at a time. I bathed the child, administered care, etc. Then, I would go home. I was on call for medical emergencies only and made this clear.

I had known from what the parents told me during my interview that the child had gone through many nurses over the course of a year. It didn't take long to figure out why.

A few times, the patient's mother texted me, asking if I could stop by a fast food place and bring them dinner, because she 'just didn't have time to cook' that day. She would ask me to pick up dry cleaning, or to run to the store for her. I always told her no, and she would be bitter for a bit, but she eventually got over it.

One day, I was bathing the patient and heard a lot of ruckus downstairs. I was finishing up in the bathroom, with the patient cradled in my arms, when his young siblings entered the bathroom and told me they were hungry.

I told them that my job was to care for their brother.

"But my mom said you'd make us lunch," one of the kids said. "She said you have to do what we tell you to do because she pays you."

"Well," I said, trying to be as nice as possible, "you can go downstairs and tell your mom that I'm a nurse, not a nanny."

"My mom's not home," the child replied.

Oh hell no.

My patient's mother had left to go shopping, leaving me with her children. All my calls to her went to voicemail. I didn't have the father's cell phone information, but I knew where he worked, so I called the main office and requested him. It took 20 minutes of being passed from multiple departments to reach him.

When I did reach him and explained the situation, he sounded like I was annoying him with my complaints. He said, "Look, you're getting paid, so what does it matter? She's usually only gone a few hours."

He hung up on me, and when I called back, his secretary told me he was no longer accepting calls.

I didn't know what else to do, so I stayed with the kids until the mother came home (five hours later, after I'd already been there two hours). The mother was mad at me because, "Oh, you fed them peanut butter sandwiches? Why couldn't you make them chicken tenders or something?"

I couldn't help it, I really couldn't. I flipped out and told the mother that what she had done was highly inappropriate. She had the gall to basically repeat what her husband and children had told me.

I told the lady, "No wonder you go through so many nurses. Hire a nanny if you want to dump your kids on someone."

She reported me to my contracting agency, but they'd had enough complaints that they told me not to worry about it, and then they told her they would no longer work with her on assigning nurses to her home.

--M.Y.

New Hampshire

I was caring for a patient who was clearly rich and used to be catered to.

I was doing rounds and brought her meds and a cup of water.

She literally slapped the cup of water out of my hand and said, "Missy, don't you dare disrespect me by bringing me tap water. I already told that other girl that I will only take my medication with an organic lemon and berry smoothie."

I kind of laughed out of anger and said, "Well, we're fresh out, so it's either water or apple juice from the cafeteria."

She screamed at me and told me to go get her an effing smoothie, and she went off on this long rant about how I was worthless and stupid because I was poor and worked for the public. She said the highlight of my life would be my ability to look back and say I waited on her.

I then told her that if she didn't like the care she was receiving, she needed to take some of her money and pay for a private care provider, instead of being such a bitch.

I was written up, but I don't regret my outburst.

--T.R.

California

When I was doing home health nursing, my 86-year-old patient asked me to give her husband a handjob.

At first, I thought she was joking, so I laughed.

But then, the patient said, "Honey, it's okay. We're old enough to understand that it's just sex, not love."

I was so uncomfortable telling someone my Nana's age that I wouldn't do that.

She responded, "Is it because of money? Sweetie, go get my pocketbook and I can give you a little extra today."

I politely told the patient that sexual favors were not in my job description and asked her not to ask again. She didn't seem to understand why I was uneasy with the proposition.

--D.T.

Florida

I'm a CNA in the ER and am basically supposed to do what RNs tell me to do. This became an argument, because the CNAs thought the RNs were being unprofessional and abusive. The RNs went to supervising and somehow got the greenlight to send us home if we refused an order, which I thought was bullshit because nobody would listen to our side of the story.

Well, one day, this pregnant RN asked me to get her a cup of ice because she didn't want to get up. She flat-out told me she didn't want to get up.

I told her no, that I work for the patients, not to be an RN's waitress.

"Do you want to go home?" she asked me. "I can tell you to clock out and go home."

I really needed the job, so I went to the back and got her ice from the dispenser that we use for ice packs and to offer service to patients.

The RN took one look in the cup and said, "You know I don't like the flaky ice. Go across the street and get me ice from the soda machine."

When I told the RN no again, she told me to clock out.

I was fired the next day, because I 'compromised' patient care and safety by leaving staff short-staffed due to insubordination. I told my side of the story, but they said two RNs came forward with signed statements that said I refused to assist with patient care.

I contacted a lawyer and got a nice severance from the hospital, but I still have to explain on my résumés why I left that job, and then people look at me like I'm lying.

I'm not a mean person by any means, but I really hope that woman gets what's coming to her.

--Initials and location withheld at request

Our guys did everything we could for a residential fire, but we could not save the home.

The resident, a man in his early-40s, pestered us nonstop because he said it was our responsibility to find him a hotel. I informed the resident that he could contact the Red Cross, but he was adamant that it was our fault that his home burned. He said we 'didn't try hard enough' and nitpicked our timing and everything else.

We eventually had to have the man removed from the scene by officers because he took a swing at me.

--C.T.
Alabama

I registered this patient who was 'so sick' that she claimed she couldn't stand. She asked if she could come behind the counter and use my computer to check her Facebook account.

When I told her no, I guess she experienced a miracle, because she was suddenly pacing the lobby, yelling about how I didn't care about how she was in pain and how desperate she was to tell all her friends she was in the ER.

I asked her why she couldn't use the cell phone she had in her hand to get on Facebook, and she said, "Bitch, I'm not paying for data, when I'm already going to be paying your ass to sit there and be rude."

Whatever. She was an LBT.

--H.L.
Kentucky

A tourist was brought in because he had appendicitis. He went to emergency surgery and his wife had been sleeping in his room for two days.

On the third day, she came to my work station, handed me a bunch of paperwork from airports, and she said, "Just tell the airlines I want to reschedule our flight. I already wrote down the times and date we want to leave. Now, our reservation is up today, so I'm going to need you to try to find us a new hotel and then take our luggage from our old room to our new room."

I was dumbfounded for a moment, but I finally said flatly, "Ma'am, I'm a nurse, not a travel agent. I can direct you to a phone, if you need to call your airline and hotel."

This woman chewed me out every which way and said that she really thought people in our country were 'better than this, but she guessed she was wrong.' Her rant was racist and disgusting.

I was seething by the time she was done yelling, but I saved my energy and repeated that I could direct her to a phone, so that she could handle her travel plans on her own.

She reported me to my supervisor and said that we needed to behave more like the people at the resort at which she had been staying.

Yeah, no.

--K.J.

Jamaica

We once had a subject file a lawsuit against our station and his arresting officers, because we 'neglected' to feed or walk his dogs during his incarceration. He couldn't find someone to take care of the animals, so we called Animal Control, and the dogs were in the facility's custody until the subject was released from jail two months later. He also sued the city because they charged him boarding and care fees while they had cared for his dogs.

He lost.

Don't walk around with a pocket full of meth if you don't have someone to take care of your pets.

There, problem solved.

--Z.H.

West Virginia

<u>Well, Duh!</u>

I work for EMS and run a social media page for our community, which includes general calls dispatched via scanner, weather advisories for our area, and occasionally generic health tips.

Following our area's first big winter storm, I posted the following:

'With the kids off from school, and the flu spreading, today is a good day to disinfect! Parents, try using Lysol and/or bleach to wipe down backpacks, lunch pails, toys, and everything your child touches inside. (Don't forget to do the same for things you touch!) Wash all backpacks and clothing, especially hats and jackets. For healthier kids and parents, use Lysol and/or bleach to kill all the bad germs!'

The weather was obviously crappy, so I decided to go back to bed for a while. I even turned my phone off because I didn't want to be interrupted by anyone for any reason.

When I woke up and turned my phone on, I had received dozens of notifications. My social media post had hit some nerves.

Apparently, some parents claimed to have used cleaning products *on* their children and themselves. One parent threatened to sue me because she sprayed Lysol on her kid's tongue and 'was angrily writing from the ER.' Some people said they used bleach wipes on themselves or sprayed Lysol on their skin and were simply writing to know how long it took for the germs to die that way.

I had to go back to my original post to include additional information: DO NOT USE CLEANING PRODUCTS ON YOURSELF OR YOUR CHILDREN. THESE PRODUCTS WARN AGAINST DOING THIS, AND I REFUSE TO BE HELD RESPONSIBLE IF YOU DO SOMETHING LIKE THIS.

This warning brought on some laughs by people who couldn't believe others could lack basic common sense, but it also landed me in hot water by all the sensitives out there, who started bashing me because "Well, you didn't make yourself clear the first time."

I was so mad. How could anyone take that out on me?

Whatever happened to people knowing not to do stupid things like that?

--B.P.

Illinois

A Message to Readers (Including a Timely Rant)

Hey, guys! It's been a while, hasn't it? Sorry for the delay, but I took the month of December 'off' from writing, hoping to clear my head and take a nice 'staycation.' If you're not familiar with that term, it basically means I stayed home and did nothing but play video games and watch TV because I'm poor and don't like being around people (ha!).

I think I touched down on this before, but as I read this material, I wanted to say it again. I don't know what I'm getting myself into when I open a message or e-mail. Sometimes, I'll be able to get a feel for the mood of a submission by the first few words I can see in the preview, or by the subject line. Otherwise, I open these communications blindly. This means that some submissions are used right away, and others are set aside (either for future books or declined for use due to their subject matter). I usually spend a few hours going through submissions when I do get around to that. There are times that I have so many non-related submissions that I don't know if they belong in the same book. Then, like you probably have noticed, I open and receive so many messages regarding the same theme that I can easily come up with a title. It wasn't my intention to write so much about foreign bodies in rectums, but I work with what I get from you guys.

I want to thank you for all your support, and I'm glad to see some new faces on Twitter and Facebook!

Okay, guys. I'm using this time to rant for a minute. I'm sure I'll catch all holy hell for it, too. <u>When I'm wrapping it up, I'll start that sentence in bold, in case you want to just skip over all this.</u>

Working in the medical field (or retired from), we see *a lot* of stupid people doing even dumber things. It's fun to joke around and say, "That's job security."

Can we not stop for a second and ask, "Who the hell didn't teach you not to eat

LAUNDRY SOAP?" (A Twitter follower also shared a link of a child snorting detergent!)

I mean, kids will be kids. One time, in high school Home Ec., we paid a guy $5 to drink a glass of water mixed with Dawn dish soap. You know what happened? He puked all over the place and our teacher spent the rest of the hour yelling at us. You know what we did? Well, we sure didn't drink water mixed with dish soap, because we all just watched what happened to that kid. I think there's a difference between, 'I bet you won't do that shit again,' and 'PSA: Please, please, PLEASE tell your kids to stop eating laundry detergent and videoing the results.'

Maybe the internet has been a great tool in assisting these asinine acts to go viral, but ultimately, we are to blame because we give these people so much attention that everyone's out to try the next craziest thing. We've seemed to have lost a little bit of our common sense, hoping to fill it with attention and grandeur as a replacement. We'd rather disrespect someone for five minutes of fame than understand that we have to live with the consequences of being an asshole for the rest of our lives.

The truth is, I can't watch the news or scroll through social media without losing faith in humanity and our future as a competent society. We very rarely see anyone practicing personal responsibility anymore, we have lost our ability to communicate civilly, and we are quick to chase people miles just to cut out their throats, rather than we're willing to meet in the middle. We're no longer entitled to personal opinions. You can't say or do anything without someone being offended or screaming at you about how wrong you are.

I have received plenty of hate mail and sour remarks about the content of my books. Bleeding hearts write hate-filled messages to me, but they'll think it's acceptable to tell a stranger, "I hope you die of cancer." I use dark humor. I'm judgmental. I know my flaws and have my demons. Some, I work on and try to get rid of. Others, they're fun, so we've joined sides. (I've yet to meet anyone without faults, but I guess all these people bashing me and everyone else for every little thing are saintly.) I won't apologize for saying what many of us think or even what I think, and I won't ask any of you to, either. I welcome all discussion and viewpoints unless you're being openly violent and/or blatantly disrespectful. Then, it becomes clear that there's no room for discussion because nothing we say to each other can diffuse the bomb in the center of the room.

I'm not sure how we ended up here. When we were growing up, remember how we used to have petty disagreements with our friends all the time?

"I want to play Dig Dug."

"Dig Dug is dumb."

"You're dumb."

Try to have that conversation in today's society, and you're going to receive death threats because you don't like Dig Dug and you're calling people dumb.

We've lost our ability to communicate while agreeing to disagree, which is a fundamental component of a peaceful way of life. Now, do I think we have problems to fix? Absolutely. I will not stand for anyone being threatened, physically harmed, or treated unequally. But I think we've forgotten that you can dislike me and what I stand for, and I can dislike you and what you stand for, but that doesn't mean that we don't owe it to each other—as human beings—to treat each other with respect. I think we all need to remember that before we hop behind a keyboard or jump in someone's face and start vilifying someone for doing or saying something we may find distasteful. There can be a middle ground.

That rant is over. Thank you for reading through that, if you did. I just couldn't sit back and watch all the things being thrown around, without speaking my mind.

You have all been wonderful readers, and again, I cannot express how much I appreciate you.

Please, with everything going on in the world today, be careful. Stay safe. And have a great day!

Check me out on Twitter!

https://twitter.com/AuthorKerryHamm

You can also find me on Facebook, by searching for 'Author Kerry Hamm.'

www.ingramcontent.com/pod-product-compliance
Lightning Source LLC
Chambersburg PA
CBHW071251220526
45468CB00001B/79